RESISTANCE BAND
WORKOUTS
FOR SENIORS

T0145984

RESISTANCE BAND
WORKOUTS
FOR SENIORS

STRENGTH TRAINING
AT HOME OR ON THE GO

KARINA INKSTER, MA, PTS
PHOTOS BY JOHN C. WATSON

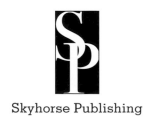

Skyhorse Publishing

Skyhorse Publishing books may be purchased in bulk at special discounts for sales promotion, corporate gifts, fund-raising, or educational purposes. Special editions can also be created to specifications. For details, contact the Special Sales Department, Skyhorse Publishing, 307 West 36th Street, 11th Floor, New York, NY 10018 or info@skyhorsepublishing.com.

Skyhorse® and Skyhorse Publishing® are registered trademarks of Skyhorse Publishing, Inc.®, a Delaware corporation.

Visit our website at www.skyhorsepublishing.com.

10 9 8 7 6 5 4 3 2

Library of Congress Cataloging-in-Publication Data is available on file.

Cover design by Daniel Brount and David Ter-Avanesyan
Cover photos by John C. Watson
Edited by Leah Zarra

Print ISBN: 978-1-5107-7010-2
Ebook ISBN: 978-1-5107-7011-9

Printed in China

CONTENTS

Introduction

If you want to improve your strength and body composition without a gym membership, this book is for you. You'll be able to work out at home, outdoors, and while traveling. My fitness coaching clients have performed their resistance band strength workouts everywhere from airports and long-haul flights, to sailboats, empty conference rooms at the office, campgrounds in the forest, and everywhere in between!

In this book, you'll discover the benefits of strength training for older adults, and the benefits of working with resistance bands in particular. You'll learn how to choose resistance bands, and how to safely use them to increase your strength. I'll go over the three types of resistance bands so you can put together your own inexpensive gym that fits into a small bag.

A collection of fifty strength exercises that work all the major muscle groups will inspire you to create—and maintain—a regular strength training practice. Once you're familiar with these exercises, you'll learn how to put together your own workout programs. After all, having fifty exercises to choose from is well and good, but they won't be of any use unless you implement them!

Strength training—also called resistance training—is one of the most effective ways of improving your body composition, preventing injuries, increasing your bone density, revving up your metabolism, and improving your day-to-day functioning. Given these wide-ranging benefits, everyone, at any age, should be strength training!

The most common form of strength training is lifting weights at a gym. However, not everyone enjoys going to gyms, and not everyone has access to these facilities. My team and I work with clients all over the world, some of whom live in extremely remote places, like the middle of Outback Australia or a tiny island in Bermuda with only twenty houses and no roads. These places certainly don't have gyms! Other clients have family responsibilities like caring for older parents or full-time care of young grandchildren, and must strength train at home. Some want to save money by not purchasing gym memberships, and others prefer training at home for logistical reasons like saving time traveling to and from a gym, or being able to fit in a quick midday strength training session while working from home.

This is where resistance bands come in. If you want to work out wherever you like, including at home and while traveling, resistance bands are the most effective, most user-friendly choice.

As more and more people learn about the incredible benefits of strength training, more and more types of exercise equipment are being produced. The options can be overwhelming! Rest assured that the humble resistance band is one of the most effective, well-studied, economical, and travel-friendly equipment options available. Professional athletes from countless different disciplines have been using resistance bands in their training for decades, especially when traveling.

This book contains everything you need to learn a wide variety of resistance band strength exercises, and put them together into a fun and effective workout program you can perform anywhere.

Benefits of Strength Training

Strength training is a form of physical exercise that uses resistance to induce muscle contraction. This builds the strength, size, and endurance of our muscles. Strength training has incredible benefits for youth and adults of all ages, including injury prevention, improved athletic performance, increased bone density, lowering our risk for many chronic diseases, and improving our day-to-day functioning.

Strength training (also called resistance training; I use the terms interchangeably) is a broad term that refers to any type of exercise that uses some form of resistance to strengthen and build muscle. We can create this resistance by using dumbbells, barbells, weight and cable machines at the gym, kettlebells, medicine balls, our own body weight, and—of course—resistance bands.

Note that when we talk about endurance within the context of strength training, we mean *anaerobic* endurance, where our muscles are relying on stored reserves of fuel, rather than oxygen. Anaerobic (without oxygen) activities are high-intensity and short duration, like sprinting or performing a challenging set of ten weighted squats.

In contrast, *aerobic* endurance refers to the ability of our respiratory and cardiovascular systems to maintain moderate-intensity exercise over extended periods. Aerobic activities involve oxygen in our muscles' energy-generating process. Swimming, jogging, or cycling at a consistent pace for thirty to sixty minutes, for example, requires aerobic endurance.

Here are some of the benefits of maintaining a consistent strength training practice. You'll reap these benefits regardless of the equipment you use—whether it's resistance bands, dumbbells, kettlebells, barbells, your own body weight, or a combination of these.

BONE DENSITY

Bone density is the amount of calcium and other minerals in our bones. Stronger, healthier bones have a higher mineral content, while low mineral content (and thus low bone density) is a risk factor for osteoporosis and bone fractures.

Bone density decreases as a normal part of aging. The good news is you can prevent and slow down this bone loss by strength training regularly! We can even build new bone in later life by resistance training consistently.[1,2] This greatly reduces our risk for osteoporosis, and improves our odds of maintaining independence in later life.

Strength training can increase bone mineral density at any age, and at any fitness level. One study found a 6 percent increase in hip bone mineral density in older women (mean age 71.9) with decreased muscle strength, after strength training for an hour, three days a week for sixteen weeks.[3] In another study, postmenopausal women with low or very low bone density improved the strength of their bones by resistance training twice a week for thirty minutes, for eight months.[4]

Other research looked at the effects of strength training in older male sprint athletes. For twenty weeks, half the study participants engaged in a strength training program along with their sprint training, and the other half continued with their regular running-based sprint training.

---

1   E. A. Marques, J. Mota, J. Carvalho. "Exercise effects on bone mineral density in older adults: a meta-analysis of randomized controlled trials," (2012): 1493–1515. https://www.ncbi.nlm.nih.gov/pmc/articles/PMC3528362.

2   G. A. Kelley, K. S. Kelley, W. M. Kohrt. "Exercise and bone mineral density in premenopausal women: a meta-analysis of randomized controlled trials," *International Journal of Endocrinology*, (2013) https://www.ncbi.nlm.nih.gov/pubmed/23401684.

3   V. Huovinen et al. "Bone mineral density is increased after a 16-week resistance training intervention in elderly women with decreased muscle strength," *European Journal of Endocrinology, 175*(6) (2016): 571–582. https://eje.bioscientifica.com/view/journals/eje/175/6/571.xml#affiliation1.

4   Watson, et al. "High-Intensity Resistance and Impact Training Improves Bone Mineral Density and Physical Function in Postmenopausal Women With Osteopenia and Osteoporosis: The LIFTMOR Randomized Controlled Trial," *Journal of Bone and Mineral Research, 34*(3) (2017): 572. https://asbmr.onlinelibrary.wiley.com/doi/full/10.1002/jbmr.3284.

The group that engaged in strength training improved the structure and strength of their tibia (shin) bones, while the tibias of those not performing strength training remained unchanged. The researchers concluded, "Intensive strength and sprint training improves mid-tibia structure and strength in middle-aged and older male sprint athletes, suggesting that in the presence of high-intensity loading exercise, the adaptability of the bone structure is maintained during aging."[5]

Weight loss can, unfortunately, be accompanied by bone mineral loss. This can happen for many reasons, including calorie restriction and not taking in enough bone-building nutrients, and a lower body weight and thus less weight-bearing work your bones have to do. If you're working on losing weight (especially a significant amount of weight), you'll need to be extra careful about maintaining your bone density.

In one randomized controlled trial lasting five months, researchers had overweight and obese participants with a mean age of sixty-nine consume a calorie-restricted diet. Half the participants engaged in resistance training (three days a week of eight upper- and lower-body strength exercises), and the other half engaged in aerobic training (four days a week of treadmill walking, while their heart rates were monitored). Lumbar spine bone mineral density remained unchanged in both groups. In the aerobic training group, hip bone density decreased slightly, while it remained the same in the resistance training group. The researchers concluded that "performing resistance, rather than aerobic, training during calorie restriction may attenuate loss of hip bone mineral density in overweight and obese older adults."[6]

---

5   T. H. Suominen et al. "Effects of a 20-week high-intensity strength and sprint training program on tibial bone structure and strength in middle-aged and older male sprint athletes: a randomized controlled trial," *Osteoporosis International, 28*(9), (2017): 2663–2673. https://link.springer.com/article/10.1007/s00198-017-4107-z.

6   K. M. Beavers et al. "Change in bone mineral density during weight loss with resistance versus aerobic exercise training in older adults," *The Journals of Gerontology: Series A, 72*(11) (2017): 1582–1585. https://academic.oup.com/biomedgerontology/article/72/11/1582/3098957.

MUSCLE MASS, STRENGTH, AND HEALTHY AGING

Strength training is about as close as you can get to a real-life "fountain of youth." Muscle mass naturally decreases as we age, but we can prevent much of this by making sure we engage in regular resistance training.

Muscle mass—particularly of the lower body—in older adults is a strong predictor of falls, mobility, and independence. One recent study found that low muscle mass in a group of more than 1,000 older adults was significantly associated with a higher fall risk ten years after being measured. In addition, low handgrip strength was associated with a higher bone fracture risk, and when body mass was taken into account, low muscle mass was associated with a higher mortality rate.[7]

Another study found that adults aged eighty and older with significant muscle loss were more than three times more likely to fall during a follow-up period of two years, compared to participants who didn't have as much muscle loss. This relationship persisted even when variables like gender, age, physical activity, number of medications, cognitive impairment, and body mass index were controlled for.[8]

Several studies have examined strength training with resistance bands. One randomized controlled trial studied overweight older women with sarcopenia (low muscle mass). After training with resistance bands for twelve weeks, participants had increased muscle mass, muscle quality, and physical function.[9] Another study found "improved muscle strength and endurance, cardiovascular function, and gait speed" in older adults with

7   S. Balogun et al. "Prospective associations of low muscle mass and function with 10-year falls risk, incident fracture and mortality in community-dwelling older adults," *The Journal of Nutrition, Health & Aging, 21*(7) (2017): 843–848. https://link.springer.com/article/10.1007/s12603-016-0843-6.

8   F. Landi et al. "Sarcopenia as a risk factor for falls in elderly individuals: Results from the ilSIRENTE study," *Clinical Nutrition, 31*(5) (2012): 652–658. https://www.sciencedirect.com/science/article/pii/S0261561412000362.

9   C. D. Liao et al. "Effects of elastic band exercise on lean mass and physical capacity in older women with sarcopenic obesity: A randomized controlled trial," *Scientific Reports, 8*(1) (2018): 2317. https://www.nature.com/articles/s41598-018-20677-7.

dementia after they trained with resistance bands three times a week for five months.[10]

A study published in the *Journal of Strength and Conditioning Research* had its participants strength train with resistance bands twice daily, five days a week, for twelve weeks. All participants were female and had Type 2 diabetes. At the end of the study, participants' blood glucose levels, body composition, and physical function had improved significantly. The researchers were investigating potential differences in training effects between women who had been recently diagnosed with diabetes and those who had long-term diabetes. They concluded, "These data suggest that patients with a long history of diabetes respond positively to resistance training and in a manner comparable to their recently diagnosed counterparts. Therefore, current inactivity in patients with long-standing disease should not deter from beginning an exercise program."[11]

A 2021 meta-analysis examined the effects of resistance band training on physical and psychological dimensions among frail older adults. The researchers analyzed fifteen studies, and found that regular resistance band exercise reduced frailty after twenty-four weeks, and reduced depression after both twelve and twenty-four weeks.[12]

Most resistance band strength training studies have focused on older populations, especially those with specific conditions like diabetes, dementia, or low muscle mass. Most participants in studies like these were sedentary before beginning the study interventions. We need a greater body

---

10 N. Ahn and K. Kim "Effects of an elastic band resistance exercise program on lower extremity muscle strength and gait ability in patients with Alzheimer's disease," *Journal of Physical Therapy Science*, *27*(6) (2015): 1953–1955. https://www.ncbi.nlm.nih.gov/pubmed/26180356.

11 B. Park et al. "Effects of Elastic Band Resistance Training on Glucose Control, Body Composition, and Physical Function in Women With Short- vs. Long-Duration Type-2 Diabetes," *Journal of Strength and Conditioning Research*, *30*(6) (2016): 1688–1699. https://www.ingentaconnect.com/content/wk/jsc/2016/00000030/00000006/art00026.

12 I. D. Saragih et al. "Effects of resistance bands exercise for frail older adults: A systematic review and meta-analysis of randomised controlled studies," *Journal of Clinical Nursing*, (July 2021), online ahead of print. https://onlinelibrary.wiley.com/doi/10.1111/jocn.15950.

of research on other populations, including younger people and those who are already active. However, given the results we've seen from other forms of strength training (as well as my and countless other coaches' experience with our clients), training with resistance bands has many of the same benefits as training with other equipment like barbells, dumbbells, and kettlebells—at any stage of the life cycle.

FAT LOSS AND BODY COMPOSITION

Improving body composition means decreasing fat and increasing muscle. In the previous section, we saw that strength training with resistance bands can help to increase muscle mass. This is an important piece of the equation, but many people also want to work on fat loss.

When it comes to body composition and changing your physique, four main factors will affect your results. In order of importance, here's what will most affect your physique:

1. *Nutrition*. Eating a diet that supports your fitness and physique goals is the foundation of getting the results you want. You may have heard the saying, "You can't out-train a bad diet!" We tend to overestimate the calories we've burned while working out, and underestimate the calories we're consuming in our food. For example, the average person would need to run one mile to burn the energy equivalent of just ten almonds.

   If you're looking to change your physique, try to view food as an athlete would: it's fuel for your training and recovery, rather than something you've "earned" after a workout (although treats, in moderation, should be a part of any long-term approach to nutrition!).

   Ensure you're eating mostly whole foods, cooking most of your meals at home, and eating an overall volume of food that suits your goals. If you're working on losing fat, you'll need to be in a calorie deficit (consuming fewer calories than you burn in a day), and if you're working on gaining muscle mass, you'll need to eat in a calorie surplus (consuming more calories than you burn in a day).

If you're strength training regularly, make sure you're consuming enough protein. Our bodies use protein to build and repair tissues, and it's a crucial building block of muscle, bone, cartilage, and skin. Protein intake is also important if you're in a calorie deficit (i.e., your physique goal is to lose fat). Ensuring you consume adequate protein will help you preserve muscle, rather than potentially lose muscle along with fat.

There is no universal recommended daily amount for protein, so individual needs will differ. Most of my clients who strength train aim to get about 20 percent of their total calories from protein. If you're active, in a healthy weight range, and looking to lose fat and/or gain muscle, aiming for 0.8–1 gram of protein per pound of body weight per day is a great place to start. For example, if you weigh 150 pounds you'd need between 120 and 150 grams of protein per day, and for a body weight of 200 pounds you'd need between 160 and 200 grams of protein per day.

2. *Strength training.* After nutrition, consistent strength training is the next important factor in physique change—and maintaining that change once you've achieved it. Many people assume that cardiovascular training will have the biggest effect on changing their physiques. Cardio can certainly play a part, especially if fat loss is your goal, but strength training gives you much more bang for your buck.

Strength training, including working out with resistance bands, is much more effective than cardio at building muscle. Since muscle is more metabolically active than fat (i.e., our bodies require more energy to maintain muscle compared to maintaining fat), the more muscle you have, the more energy you'll burn on a daily basis—even when you're not working out.

When people talk about wanting to achieve a "toned" look, what they mean is building muscle and losing fat. Muscles do two things: they shrink when they're not used, or they grow when they're challenged. The concept of "toning" means developing muscle, and then losing fat, if necessary, to reveal it. Cardio can help you lose fat, but it won't build much muscle.

Ideally, your workout routine would involve both strength training and cardio. Make strength training your priority, and fit in cardio when you can. My own weekly training schedule, for example, includes five 45-minute strength training sessions, with a 10- or 15-minute jump rope session after one of them, plus three 30-minute swim workouts and a hike most weekends.

3. *Sleep and recovery*. Proper recovery is essential to making progress with your strength and physique. Tissue repair and muscle growth happen mostly while we sleep, so it's important to prioritize getting enough shut-eye. Put another way: your muscles don't get stronger while you're training. They get stronger while you're sleeping!

   On page 159 you'll find more information on recovering from your workouts.

4. *Cardio and conditioning*. The "cherry on top" of the physique change hierarchy is cardio and conditioning. As mentioned, cardiovascular activity can help you lose fat, although it'll have a smaller overall impact compared to your nutrition. Cardio is important for heart and lung health, and having good cardiovascular conditioning can help you to recover more quickly from strength training sets.

   Conditioning typically combines strength with cardio, and usually involves anaerobic (high intensity, short duration) activity.

   The US Office of Disease Prevention and Health Promotion and the Canadian Society for Exercise Physiology both recommend, for all adults, a minimum of 150 minutes of moderate- to vigorous-intensity aerobic exercise each week, in bouts of 10 minutes or more.

STRENGTH TRAINING RECOMMENDATIONS

In addition to the aerobic exercise we should perform each week, the US Office of Disease Prevention and Health Promotion and the Canadian Society for Exercise Physiology recommend, for all adults, a minimum of two strength training sessions per week, working all your major muscle groups each time.

These organizations add that those adults aged sixty-four and older with poor mobility should "perform physical activities to enhance balance and prevent falls," and that for all adults, "more physical activity provides greater health benefits."[13,14]

To reap the greatest rewards from strength training, I recommend aiming for three 30-minute strength training sessions per week if you're just starting out. Once you've maintained this habit for about two months, try increasing the length of your workouts to forty-five minutes.

Then, if your schedule allows, you can also increase your training to four days per week, working upper body and lower body on alternating days, rather than all your major muscle groups in each workout. See the sample workout programs on page 145 to learn how to structure your workouts.

---

13 Canadian Society for Exercise Physiology. (2011). "Canadian Physical Activity Guidelines for Adults 18–64 years." https://www.csep.ca/CMFiles/Guidelines/CSEP _PAGuidelines_adults_en.pdf.
14 US Office of Disease Prevention and Health Promotion. "Physical Activity Guidelines for Americans." https://health.gov/dietaryguidelines/2015/guidelines/appendix-1.

BEFORE YOU START STRENGTH TRAINING

If you have a condition like arthritis, osteoporosis, or high blood pressure, make sure that your doctor has given you the go-ahead to start a strength training program. If you're getting into resistance training for the first time, to ensure you're using correct form, I recommend working with a fitness professional until you're confident you can perform each movement effectively and safely. I provide detailed instructions and photos in this book for you to learn each movement, but an extra set of trained eyes can always help! Taking video clips of yourself performing strength exercises, then comparing the clips to the photos in this book, can be an effective method of checking your own form.

When you're performing the exercises in this book, make sure your movement is controlled at all times. You want to feel resistance in both directions of each movement, instead of letting the elastic snap back under its own force (this would be the equivalent of letting a dumbbell quickly drop back down toward the ground, instead of guiding it, slowly, using your muscles).

THE IMPORTANCE OF CONSISTENT TRAINING

I'm often asked by clients how long it will take to get a certain result, whether it's fat loss, improved cardiovascular conditioning, or strength and muscle gains. My answer is always the same: "I have no idea." Results will vary—greatly. Even between people following the exact same program. That's just how body types, genetics, and individual differences work.

I'd like to remind you of three things, all of which I learned over the last twenty years of strength training regularly:

1. A "transformation" might take longer than you think.
In an industry rife with ads for jaw-dropping, clickbait-worthy physique

"transformations" that supposedly take only a few weeks to accomplish, keep in mind that most real, lasting results (that don't involve unmaintainable, drastic, and/or unhealthy dieting or training plans) generally take a long time to achieve. That's not a bad thing; it's extra incentive to make healthy, active living a lifelong habit.

In general, a reasonable time frame for getting really noticeable results (both performance-wise and physique-wise) is years, not weeks or months.

The faster you get results, the easier it is to lose them. It usually means you've done something drastic and unmaintainable that has an end date. Your results, too, then automatically have an end date. Telling you that it can take a long time to get results isn't meant to discourage you. It's meant as a reality check, and as encouragement to keep going.

2. Consistency, consistency, consistency.

It doesn't sound flashy or exciting, but consistency is the best predictor of getting results. Slow and steady really is the way to win the (proverbial) race. Focus on making your active lifestyle enjoyable, sustainable, and life-enhancing—all in the name of consistency.

Over the past twenty years I focused on building maintainable habits that I could be consistent with. I didn't do anything drastic, and I didn't do anything I couldn't maintain long-term. No quick fixes, no major fluctuations in fitness or physique, just steadily creating a new normal. I've added up small habits, all of which I intend to keep for life.

Because I built my health and fitness habits slowly and sustainably, my fitness and physique don't change throughout the year, other than the slow and cumulative improvements from training, of course. There's nothing wrong with having different training seasons (e.g., a summer cardio sport or competition season, and a winter "bulking" or strength training season), but since my preferred activity is strength training, I train similarly year-round. I don't have to worry about losing the strength and muscle gains I've made, because my habits aren't going to change. And that was the whole point of starting this lifestyle in the first place: your training and your nutrition need to be a part of your life, not something you do in order to have the life you want later.

3. People who succeed in achieving their long-term goals don't stay on the health and fitness bandwagon 100 percent of the time. Everyone falls off once in a while. What separates those who get results from those who don't is the people who keep getting back on.

In my work with clients, I'll often come across the "all or nothing" mindset. It's a pattern of behavior in which someone feels they've made a small lapse in their healthy eating or regular physical activity habits, and assume that their whole practice is now shot. The entire practice gets abandoned, and exactly zero results are created. We need to find ways of outsmarting our own brains and moving away from this pattern.

At some point, every single person is going to fall off the health and fitness bandwagon for one reason or another, either for self-imposed reasons, or those beyond our control. We get sick, we need to care full time for an ill family member, we go on vacation, we get injured (hopefully rarely, if ever!), we go through a stressful move to the other side of the country . . . you get the idea. All that matters is getting back on the bandwagon as soon as we can.

This is just how life works! It's always going to be throwing unexpected things at you that could—and sometimes will—make you fall off your health and fitness bandwagon. Commit to a lifelong active, healthy living lifestyle, keep getting back on the bandwagon, and your small, consistent actions will lead to massive results over time.

Training with resistance bands can help you maintain a consistent, long-term exercise schedule, since you can use them anywhere! Work out at home if you can't get to the gym, pack them when you travel, or use them during the day in short bursts to break up long periods of sitting. As one of my clients recently told me when she got her first set of resistance bands, "I no longer have any excuses not to train!"

THE SCALE IS NOT A USEFUL TOOL FOR MEASURING RESULTS

For people who strength train regularly, measuring body weight is not the most effective method of tracking progress with your fitness and physique. Stepping on the scale will tell you what your body weighs, but it won't tell you what your body is made of. When strength training regularly (and accompanying this with a healthy diet), many people find that their body weight remains the same—or even increases. This can be discouraging if you're not also using other methods of body composition measurement, like taking progress photos and girth measurements. You can also get a DEXA scan, which uses x-ray technology to measure bone density and body composition (fat versus muscle).

One pound of muscle takes up much less space than one pound of fat. Many of my clients, as they start strength training for the first time, find that their body weights stay the same, but their measurements (e.g. waist, chest, hip, thigh, etc.) decrease. They're getting smaller overall, while maintaining the same weight. This is an excellent sign of having improved their body composition: more muscle, and less fat.

So, make sure you don't use the scale as your only method of physique progress measurement. Forget it altogether, or use it along with progress photos and girth measurements.

A NOTE ON WRIST PAIN

Many older adults (and younger ones, too!) experience wrist discomfort during exercises that involve supporting their body weight on one or both arms with flexed wrists. Think of the top position of a push-up, or performing a mountain climber. In both exercises, your hands are flat on the floor, arms straight, and you're supporting your body weight on your hands and toes.

If exercises like these cause wrist discomfort, try using push-up handles. They put your wrists in a neutral position, instead of flexed, which can feel more comfortable. Ensure the handles you use are padded with foam, and remain in a fixed position (one type of push-up handle rotates as you use them).

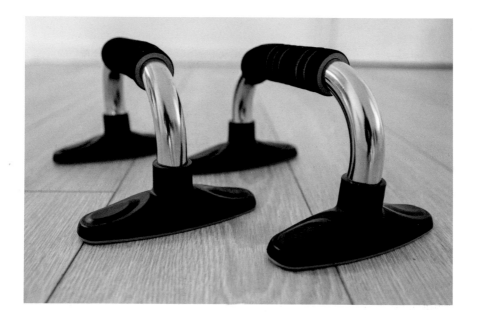

Introduction to Resistance Bands

BENEFITS OF RESISTANCE BANDS

Resistance bands are a simple way of creating external resistance that your muscles need to work against. They have many unique benefits for people of all ages and fitness levels, including those completely new to strength training, professional athletes, and everyone in between. They're inexpensive, versatile, and don't take up much space. This means you can use them to work out anywhere: at home, outdoors, or while traveling.

Resistance bands provide much more opportunity for adjusting the difficulty of exercises compared to equipment like dumbbells and barbells. Resistance bands come in different strengths (e.g., ten pounds, twenty pounds, etc.), but you can easily adjust the difficulty level of an exercise using the same band. Let's say you're using a fifteen-pound band to perform a standing row. If you step closer to your anchor point, the exercise will become easier, and if you move further away from your anchor point, the exercise will become more challenging. This allows for a lot of "fine-tuning" to occur during your sets. You can start a set standing far away from your anchor point, and move closer as needed to maintain good form. These incremental changes in difficulty can be smaller than using a dumbbell of a different weight, so you can be sure that your muscles will always be challenged at an appropriate level.

Like the workout programs I have for you in this book, resistance bands can be used on their own, or they can be combined with other pieces of equipment. Many of my clients have a few resistance bands in their gym bags, and use them for specific moves as part of their gym workouts.

They can also be useful for people with injuries or joint issues. My clients with arthritis, for example, often find resistance band handles more comfortable to hold than dumbbells, barbells, or cable machine attachments. In other cases, when someone experiences an injury or needs to recover from surgery, resistance bands can be a great interim option for strength training before getting back into dumbbell and barbell training.

Resistance bands are unique in that they offer what's called *accommodating resistance*. This means that you get a different level of resistance at the top versus the bottom of an exercise. With dumbbell, kettlebell, or barbell work, the resistance you're using stays the same throughout your exercise. When you're using equipment like this, some exercises get easier toward the end of the movement, like bench presses, overhead presses, and squats. For these movements, the weight feels heavier at the beginning of the move, and lighter at the end. This is called an ascending strength curve. With a barbell, for example, you might be able to squat 100 pounds for quarter reps, but only 60 pounds for full reps.

Other movements become more challenging toward the end of the motion, including dumbbell rows, cable machine pull-downs, seated rows, and chin-ups. These movements involve a descending strength curve. For a bent-over dumbbell row, you might be able to row a 20-pound weight halfway up, but you may need to use 12 pounds in order to perform the entire movement. Or in a pull-up you might be able to get yourself halfway up to the bar, and then need some assistance to finish the movement.

With resistance bands, the load increases as you move through an exercise's range of motion. Let's use the resistance band split squat as an example, where you're standing with your front foot on a resistance band, holding the handles at shoulder height (see page 107). At the bottom of the movement, when your legs are bent and your front thigh is parallel to the ground, you'll get the least amount of tension on the band. At the top of the movement, when both your legs are straight, you'll get the most tension on the band. This maps perfectly onto the split squat's strength curve: using a resistance band is making what is normally the easiest part of the split squat more challenging! If you were to use dumbbells instead of a resistance band, the load would not change throughout the movement.

Using bands—or adding them to barbell and/or dumbbell movements—can greatly increase your strength through a full range of motion. This is common in powerlifting training, where athletes will often add resistance bands to their deadlifts, squats, and bench presses. They can be used to increase the difficulty of the top of a movement (like the lockout position of a deadlift or squat), or to decrease the difficulty of the bottom of a movement (like the bottom of a bench press, where the barbell is lifted off the chest).

In one study, male and female college basketball, wrestling, and hockey athletes trained with barbells alone, or with barbells fitted with resistance bands. Elastic tension was accounted for so that each group was doing a similar amount of work. After seven weeks of resistance training, the group that had resistance bands added to their barbells had gained significantly more strength and power than the group that was using only barbells.[1]

WHERE YOU CAN USE RESISTANCE BANDS AND ANCHOR POINTS

Many resistance band exercises involve standing directly on the band to anchor it in place while you perform the movement. For a biceps curl, for example, you stand with both feet on a band, one handle in each hand. You then curl the handles toward your shoulders while your feet keep the band in place.

To get the most out of resistance band training and to be able to perform the greatest variety of movements, you'll need an anchor point. If you're adding resistance band exercises to your gym routine, you can

---

1   C. E. Anderson, G. A. Sforzo, J. A. Sigg. "The Effects of Combining Elastic and Free Weight Resistance on Strength and Power in Athletes," *Journal of Strength and Conditioning Research, 22*(2) (2008): 567–574.

loop a resistance band around almost any stable piece of gym equipment, like a squat rack, cable machine post, treadmill rail, or weight machine seat post. If you're using resistance bands outdoors, you'll need to find a sturdy anchor point like a small tree, fencepost, stair railing, or a piece of playground equipment (or, why not bring along a workout buddy and take turns holding the band while the other performs an exercise?).

Many of us use resistance bands at home, or while traveling. It can be difficult to find suitable anchor points in these situations. Luckily, most resistance band sets come with a door anchor, so all you need is a door, and you're set. Slide your resistance band through the loop on one end of the anchor. On the other end is a round foam stopper. Close the door with the loop on one side and the stopper on the other side, and you'll be able to perform a host of pulling and pushing movements with your resistance band.

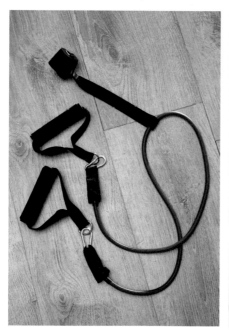
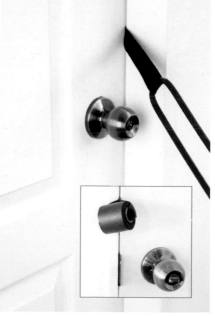

TYPES OF RESISTANCE BANDS

Tubing with handles

These are the resistance bands with which we're most familiar. Often found in commercial gyms, personal training studios, and outdoor boot-camps, they're heavy-duty lengths of elastic (sometimes covered in fabric) with handles on each end. These are the most versatile out of all resistance band options, and thus most of the exercises in this book use this type of band.

> ### What Should I Buy?
> I recommend purchasing a set of five resistance bands, each with a differ-ent resistance level, making sure that the set comes with a door anchor. This will allow you to perform a large variety of strength exercises that require looping your bands around a sturdy anchor point. A door anchor will also give you the option of performing effective hotel room workouts while traveling.
>
> Make sure the set you buy has interchangeable handles (rather than handles directly attached to each band). This way you'll be able to com-bine bands for far more resistance level options.

Mini-bands

Mini-bands are small loops of flat elastic, most commonly used for lower body training—specifically glutes—by adding resistance when looped around your ankles, shins, or knees. Most mini-bands are made out of latex, but fabric options are also available for those with latex allergies.

A greater proportion of regular resistance band (tubing with handles) exercises are for the upper body or core muscle groups compared to lower body ones, so having mini-bands available ensures you can train your legs just as much as you train your other muscle groups.

Mini-bands are also an excellent way of engaging muscles that would otherwise be difficult to target. The gluteus medius muscle, for example, is on the side of your hip and is responsible for leg abduction (moving your leg out to the side of your body). With standard barbell and dumbbell strength exercises, this muscle is difficult to target by itself. With mini-bands, however, we can train this muscle very easily by performing clam-shells, lateral walks, lying leg abductions, and more. Whenever you loop a mini-band around your legs (at your ankles, around your shins, or above your knees) and work against its resistance to keep your knees apart, you're using your gluteus medius muscles. A set of mini-bands takes up as much space as a wallet, so they're extremely convenient for travel.

What Should I Buy?
I suggest buying a set of three or four mini-bands, each with a different resistance level. Their standard circumference is between eighteen and twenty-four inches.

Superbands

"Superbands" are typically used for assisted pull-ups. That is, allowing you to do the pull-up movement without using your full body weight; the band provides assistance. These large elastic loops are typically attached to a pull-up bar, with the other end looped around your knees or feet. This way, you can learn the movement pattern of pull-ups and chin-ups, while receiving assistance from the band.

These bands, like other resistance bands, come in different resistance levels. Unlike other bands, however, they're usually standardized by color. Blue is thickest and provides the most assistance. Green is next, and is the most commonly found in commercial gyms. Then comes purple, and lastly, with the least amount of assistance, red. If you're training to do your first unassisted pull-up or chin-up, using these bands (along with other training progressions) can be very helpful. As your strength increases, you move to resistance bands with lower and lower levels of assistance.

Pull-ups and chin-ups are not the only exercises that can be done with these bands. In the exercise section of this book, you'll learn how to use them to perform five unique and challenging strength moves. You may not have seen these before!

What Should I Buy?
A set of regular resistance bands and a set of mini-bands should be your first priority. If you want to spice things up, I'd suggest getting one each of the green and purple superbands, especially if you want to work toward nailing your first pull-up!

HOW TO ADJUST RESISTANCE LEVEL/WEIGHT

Resistance bands

Most resistance bands come in sets of three to five different resistance levels. In addition to using bands of different strengths, there are three main ways to adjust the difficulty level of your resistance band exercises:

1. Combine bands. Assuming you have a resistance band set with interchangeable handles, you can use multiple bands at once to increase the difficulty level.

2. If you're performing an exercise that involves an anchor point (e.g., standing row on page 70), stand closer to the anchor point to make the move easier, and stand farther away from the anchor point to make the move more challenging.

3. If you're performing an exercise that involves standing on the resistance band (e.g., biceps curl on page 40), move your feet closer together to make the move less challenging, and move your feet farther apart to make the move more challenging.

Mini-bands

Just like regular resistance bands, mini-bands also come in a variety of different strengths. You'll need to experiment to find a level that works for you, and this might change from exercise to exercise.

Mini-bands are typically looped just above the knees, or around the ankles or shins. If you're using the heaviest strength mini-band for an exercise and it's not feeling challenging enough, add a second band over-top the first one. Another option is to add a second band around a different part of your leg. If, for example, you're performing the lateral walk exercise (see page 92) with a band around your knees, you can increase the level of difficulty by adding another band around your shins.

HOW TO CHOOSE AN APPROPRIATE RESISTANCE LEVEL

Choosing an appropriate resistance level will depend on the strength exercise you're performing, and the number of reps you're aiming for. Compound movements that require multiple muscle groups generally involve higher resistance, while isolation movements for only one muscle group at a time require less resistance. For example, a standing chest press (page 42) works the chest, shoulder, and triceps muscles simultaneously, while the pec fly (page 66) works only the chest. You'll want to use more resistance for the chest press versus the pec fly.

The most common rep range in strength training is between ten and fifteen reps. Athletes training for sheer strength, like powerlifters, will often work with lower reps and higher weights, while endurance athletes will perform some of their strength movements for higher reps. The vast majority of resistance training, however, occurs in the ten- to fifteen-rep range.

To ensure you get the most "bang for your buck" out of each set of strength exercises, make sure that the movement starts to feel very challenging *before* you've hit your target reps. For example, if you're aiming for ten reps, make sure rep number seven feels very challenging. If you're aiming for fifteen reps, make sure rep number eleven or twelve feels very challenging.

By the end of each set, you should have only one or two reps left "in the tank." There's no need to take your muscles to complete failure—where you cannot perform another rep—because you're more likely to compromise your exercise form at this point, and thus potentially injure yourself.

I often use the rate of perceived exertion (RPE) measurement with my clients. It's a 1-to-10 scale, where 1 is very little effort (sitting on the couch), and 10 is maximum effort (all-out sprinting). Your goal when you're strength training is an RPE of 7 out of 10.

Keep in mind that it doesn't matter what weights or resistance levels we use. Our muscles don't care about numbers! What matters is *effort*, and how challenging an exercise feels to you, rather than using a particular weight or resistance level.

Someone who's completely new to strength training may feel a 7 out of 10 RPE when using a ten-pound resistance band for a chest press, for example. A professional athlete may need to use a sixty-pound resistance band to get the same 7 out of 10 RPE for the same movement.

Some discomfort is inherent in strength training. Challenging our muscles isn't supposed to feel easy! However, make sure you're not feeling any "bad" pain while you're performing your workouts (e.g., a tweaked low back, knee or hip pain, etc.), and never compromise good exercise form for a higher resistance level or eking out a few extra reps.

Resistance Band Exercises

The descriptions in this section each describe one rep of an exercise. A good starting point is to aim for three sets of between ten and twelve reps per exercise, using a resistance level that feels very challenging by rep number seven. My general rule when you're aiming for ten to twelve reps is if you can perform fifteen reps with good form, the resistance level is too light. You're not just arbitrarily performing ten to twelve reps. You should be able to perform *only* ten to twelve reps, with one or two reps "left in the tank."

Never sacrifice form for increased resistance level or increased reps. Try to make each rep look the same. While your exercises should certainly feel challenging by the time you've finished each set, you should feel in control of the movement at all times.

You'll find more information on reps, sets, and designing your own workouts starting on page 135.

The exercises in this section are organized alphabetically, so you can easily find exercises included in the sample workouts section of this book. Below are the exercises organized by resistance band type (see page 21 for a description of resistance band types).

RESISTANCE BAND EXERCISES

Arnold press

Band pull-apart

Bent-over rear delt fly

Bent-over row

Biceps curl

Chest press

Face pull

Front raise

High-low chop

High curl

Incline chest press

Kickstand deadlift

Kneeling pull-down

Lateral raise

Low-high chop

Low curl

Overhead extension

Overhead press

Pallof press

Pec fly

Pull-through

Quadruped kickback

Side lunge

Side plank row

Single leg hip extension

Split squat

Standing rear delt fly

Standing row

Standing wide row

Straight arm pulldown

Torso rotation

Triceps kickback

Triceps press-down

MINI-BAND EXERCISES

Banded squat

Bicycle crunch

Clamshell

Glute bridge

Incline push-up

Lateral walk

Lying abduction

Mountain climber

Psoas march

Single leg glute bridge

SUPERBAND EXERCISES

Superband deadlift

Superband hip hinge

Superband single leg press

Superband seated row

BREATHING

For all strength training, including using resistance bands, breathing is an important part of performing each movement correctly. Breathing properly will help you to control your blood pressure while strength training (holding your breath can spike blood pressure), get as much oxygen to your muscles as possible, and perform each movement using the correct muscles and the correct form.

To ensure you're delivering as much oxygenated air as possible to your lungs, think about breathing into your belly each time you inhale.

Test your breathing: Put one hand on your chest, and the other just below your belly button. Take a deep inhalation. If you're breathing effectively, you'll feel your belly expand. If you're breathing shallowly, you'll feel your chest expand.

A useful phrase to remember is "exhale on exertion." During the concentric phase of a movement (when your muscles are contracting, like bringing your hands toward your shoulders during a biceps curl), you should be exhaling. Doing so will help you engage your core muscles as you complete the movement. Inhale during the eccentric phase of each movement (when your muscles are lengthening, like lowering your hands from your shoulders back down toward your hips during a biceps curl).

Some examples:

Squat: Inhale as you lower into a squat, and exhale as you straighten your legs back to standing.

Chest press: Exhale as you push the resistance band handles away from you, and inhale as you bring your hands back toward your chest.

Glute bridge: Exhale as you lift your hips off the floor, and inhale as you bring them back down.

PERFORMING REPS

Rather than alternating sides as we often do with dumbbell moves (e.g., reverse lunges while holding dumbbells), with resistance band moves we typically complete all reps on one side, and then switch sides and complete all reps on that side. Most often this comes down to logistics: with movements like split squats, reverse lunges, and kickstand deadlifts, for example, you have a resistance band looped under one foot. Switching sides with each rep and standing on the band with alternating feet would take up too much time and would interfere with the flow of your workout.

Tempo

To ensure you get the most out of each exercise and to prevent injury, it's important to be aware of rep tempo. Strength training tempos are often noted as four numbers, like "2-0-2-0" or "2-1-1-0." All numbers refer to seconds.

The first number describes the eccentric phase of the movement, when your muscles are lengthening. For example: lowering your hands toward the ground in a biceps curl, lowering yourself into a squat, returning to lying on the ground after performing a glute bridge, or bringing your hands from overhead back to the start position at shoulder height in an overhead press. The second number represents the number of seconds to pause at the bottom of the movement, and the third number represents the number of seconds it should take to perform the concentric portion of the exercise, where your muscles are contracting. Concentric movements include bringing your hands toward your shoulders in a biceps curl, returning to standing from a squat position, lifting your hips off the ground in a glute bridge, or pressing your hands overhead in an overhead press. The last number refers to the number of seconds to pause in the contracted position.

Let's use a squat as an example, with a "2-0-2-0" tempo. This means taking two seconds to lower into a squat, and two seconds to come back to standing, with no pausing at the lowest (squatting) and highest (standing) points of the exercise.

A "2-1-1-0" tempo for a squat would mean taking two seconds to lower until your thighs are parallel to the ground, pausing in the bottom position for one second, taking one second to press back up to standing, with no pause in the standing position.

Each resistance band exercise will vary slightly in the best tempo to use, and you'll also have personal preferences for different excrcises. In general, I'd recommend a 2-1-1-0 or 2-1-1-1 tempo for most resistance band exercises. You'd perform a biceps curl, for instance, by lowering your hands from your shoulders to the ground in two seconds, pausing with straight arms for a second, bringing your hands back to your shoulders in one second, and pausing for another second (for a 2-1-1-1 tempo). A split squat might make more sense with a 2-1-1-0 tempo: bending your legs and lowering into the split squat in two seconds, pausing at the bottom of the rep for one second, pressing back up to standing in one second, and then immediately lowering into the next rep.

UPPER BODY EXERCISES

ARNOLD PRESS

This overhead press variation targets the anterior delt (the front of your shoulder) a bit more than standard overhead presses.

Stand with both feet on a resistance band, hip width apart. Hold the handles in front of your shoulders, with your palms facing toward you. Brace your abdominal muscles (as if you were about to cough) and squeeze your glutes.

Maintaining this posture, press the band handles overhead. As you press, rotate your hands so that your palms face forward at the top of the movement, and move your hands slightly closer together. Your arms should be straight, and your biceps should be next to your ears. Reverse the movement to return to the start position.

Make sure you keep your glutes and abs activated throughout this movement to prevent hyperextending your spine, especially when you're using a challenging resistance level.

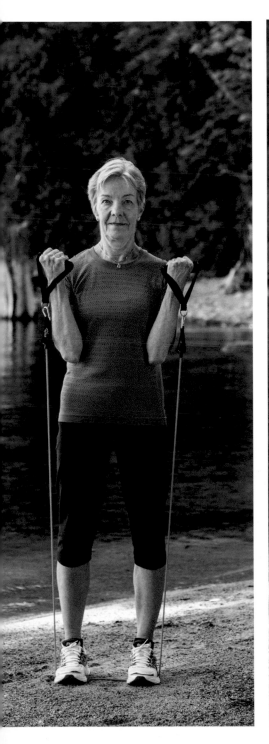
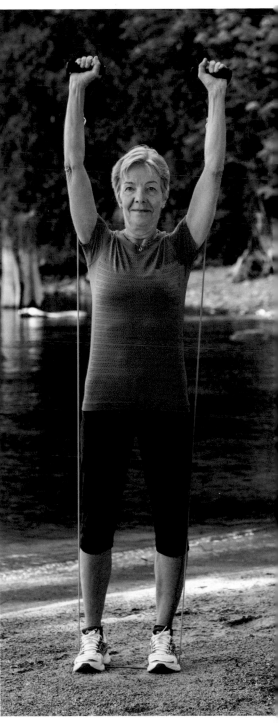

BAND PULL-APART

This is an excellent warm-up movement to perform before working on upper body exercises like push-ups, chest press, and rows. It activates your rear deltoids, which are important to overall shoulder health (and are often neglected in strength training programs).

Stand with your feet shoulder-width apart, and your spine neutral (head, torso, and hips in a stacked position). Start with your arms extended straight out in front of you at shoulder height, holding a resistance band with both hands. Your palms should be facing the floor.

Keeping your arms straight, perform a reverse fly motion, bringing your hands out laterally to your sides. Focus on activating your rear delts and upper back, bringing the band to your chest. Hold the contraction briefly, then return to the start position.

Keep your arms parallel to the ground; don't let them drop down during your set.

Move your hands closer together on the band to make this move more difficult, and move them farther away from each other to make the move less challenging.

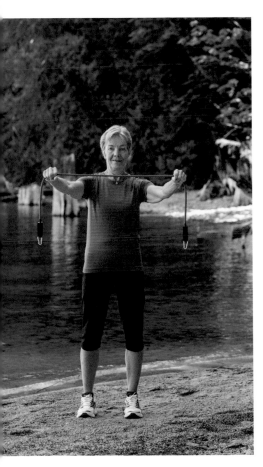
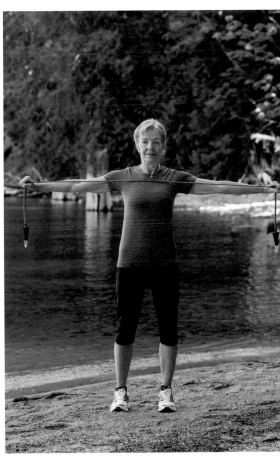

BENT-OVER REAR DELT FLY

This is a variation of the standing rear delt fly, and a good option when you don't have an anchor point to use.

Stand with both feet on a resistance band, holding a handle in each hand. Hinge your hips back behind you and bend your torso forward, keeping your spine neutral and your head in line with your spine.

Start with your arms straight toward the ground, with a slight bend in your elbows. Raise your arms out to the side, squeezing your shoulder blades together. Bring your arms parallel to the floor, pause briefly, then slowly return to the start position.

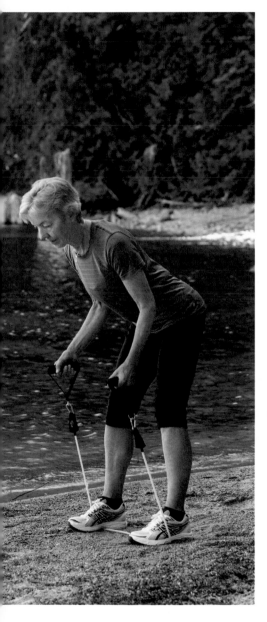

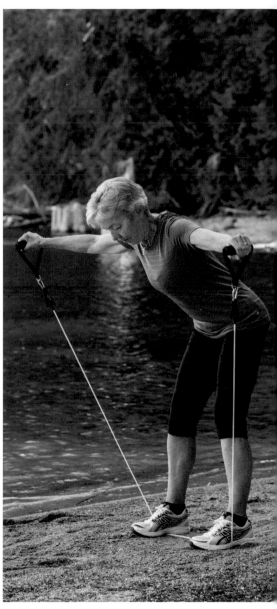

BENT-OVER ROW

This exercise mimics one of the most important upper body dumbbell strength exercises, working all the major muscles of the back.

Stand with both feet on a resistance band. Cross the handles so you're holding the right handle in your left hand, and the left handle in your right hand. Hinge your hips back behind you and bend your torso forward, keeping your spine neutral and your head in line with your spine.

Start with your arms straight toward the ground. If you don't feel tension on the band in this position, pull some slack out of the band between your feet, and/or stand with your feet farther apart.

Row the band handles upward to each side of your chest, squeezing your shoulder blades together as you row. Hold the contracted position for a second, then lower your arms to the start position.

To protect the health of your shoulders, make sure your elbows come to just past your torso, rather than moving farther back behind you and pointing toward the ceiling in the top position of the movement.

For back-strengthening movements like this one, try holding the resistance band handles with a loose grip, focusing on using your back muscles to pull the band, rather than your hands.

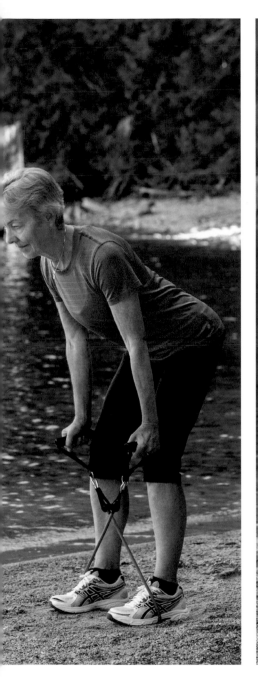
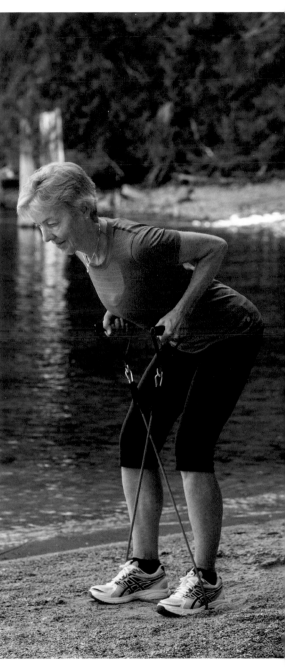

BICEPS CURL

This isolation movement targets the biceps, the muscle group on the front of your arms.

Stand on a resistance band with your feet hip width apart, holding a handle in each hand, knees slightly bent. With your palms facing forward, pin your elbows to your sides, keep your shoulders down and away from your ears, and squeeze your shoulder blades together.

Keeping your wrists in a neutral position (hands in line with your forearms), bring your hands toward your shoulders. Pause briefly, then return to the start position. Avoid the tendency to curl your wrists toward you as you bring the resistance band handles toward your shoulders.

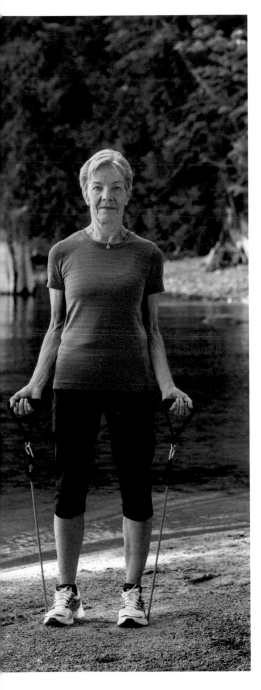 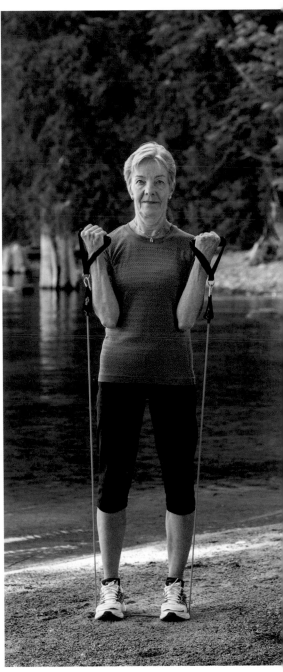

CHEST PRESS

This exercise strengthens your pectorals (chest muscles), triceps, and anterior deltoids (front of the shoulder), the same muscles that are involved in performing push-ups and bench presses.

Stand facing away from your anchor point, set to about chest height. Start with each side of the band under your arms, with your hands to the outside of your chest. You can stand with your feet hip width apart and knees slightly bent, or in a split stance with one foot in front of the other (I find the latter option more stable when using heavy resistance).

Press the resistance band handles out in front of you, bringing your hands closer together (but not touching) near the end of the movement. This mimics a dumbbell bench press movement, in which you'd start with dumbbells on either side of your chest, bringing them to almost touching as you extend your arms.

Bring your hands back to the start position, and repeat for reps.

As you start using heavier resistance levels, you may find that you need to lean forward slightly so you're not pulled backward. This is perfectly fine—just make sure your torso stays in the same position throughout each set, rather than leaning backwards and forwards with each rep.

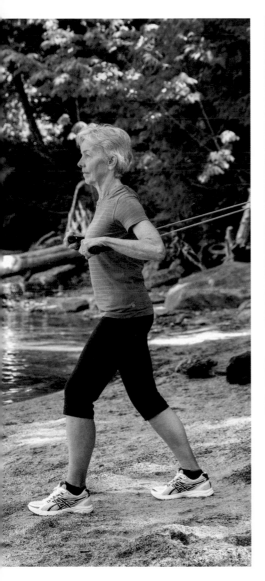
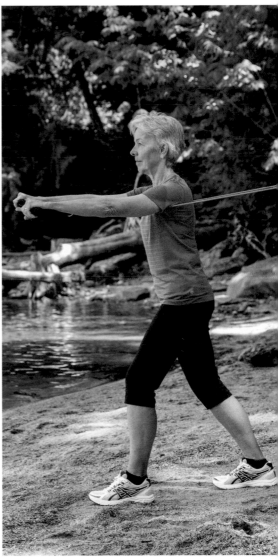

FACE PULL

The face pull is one of the most effective movements for shoulder health. It develops the posterior deltoids, which are often neglected in other shoulder exercises. This will build overall shoulder strength and prevent muscular imbalance.

Stand facing your anchor point, set to eye level. Bend your knees slightly and brace your core. Start with your arms straight, at shoulder height, with your palms facing down.

Pull the resistance band handles back and to either side of your head, squeezing your shoulder blades together as you move. Bring the handles as far back as you can without hyperextending your low back, or creating movement anywhere in your body other than your arms. Hold the contracted position briefly, then return to the start position.

Make sure you keep your shoulders down and away from your ears throughout the exercise. For back-strengthening movements like this one, try holding the resistance band handles with a loose grip, focusing on using your back muscles to pull the band, rather than your hands.

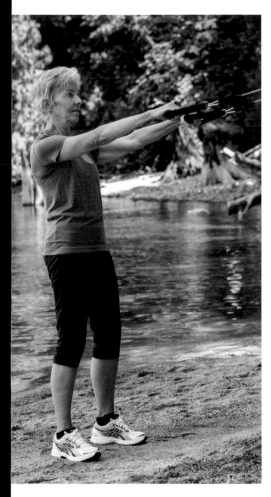
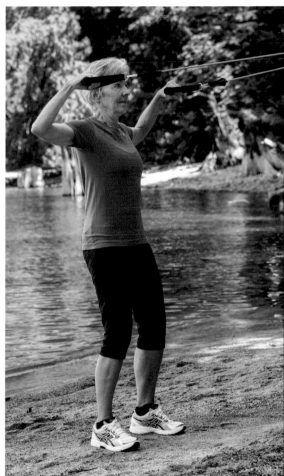

FRONT-ANCHORED REAR DELT OVERHEAD PRESS

I came across this move thanks to sports performance specialist Dr. John Rusin. As an injury prevention expert, he's created many unique exercises that simultaneously strengthen muscles and guard against injury. This is one of them, focusing on the posterior deltoids (the back of your shoulder)—a muscle group critical to posture and overall shoulder health.

Stand facing your anchor point, set to about chest height. Bend your knees slightly, and brace your core. Hold the handles in front of your shoulders, with your palms facing away from you.

Press the band handles overhead, moving your hands slightly closer together near the top of the move. Your arms should be straight, and your biceps should be next to your ears. Reverse the movement to return to the start position.

Your arms are moving in exactly the same way as they would during a "regular" overhead press. In this variation, though, the band tension is coming from the front rather than from below, so the challenge is to keep your arms from moving forward.

Make sure you keep your glutes and abs activated throughout this movement to prevent hyperextending your spine.

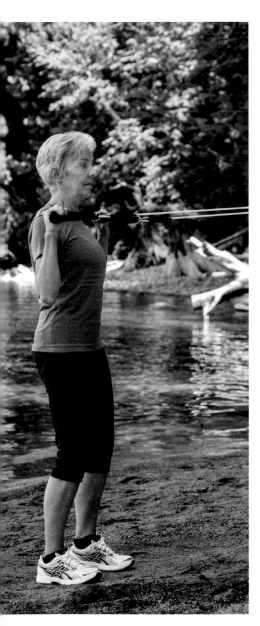
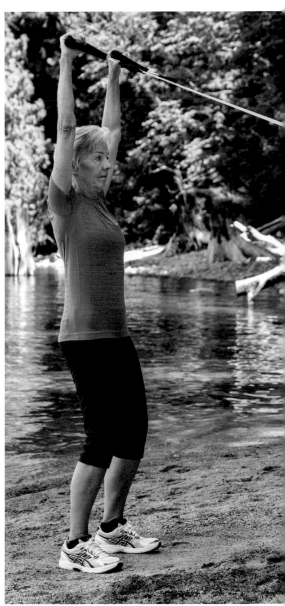

FRONT RAISE

This exercise focuses on the anterior (front) head of the shoulder muscle. Make sure you round out your shoulder training by including moves to target the other muscle heads as well, such as rear delt flys and lateral raises.

Stand with both feet on a resistance band, hands in front of your thighs and knees slightly bent. Make sure your shoulders are down and away from your ears.

Keeping your arms straight, raise your arms in front of you until they're parallel to the floor. Hold the contracted position for a second, then lower back to the start position.

Make sure you maintain perfect posture throughout the movement, with your head in line with your spine, and back neutral (not hyperextended). Avoid the tendency to lean back as you raise your arms, especially with heavier resistance levels.

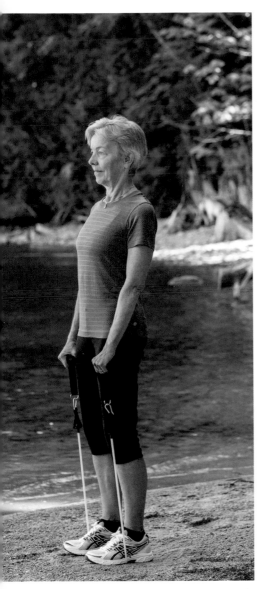
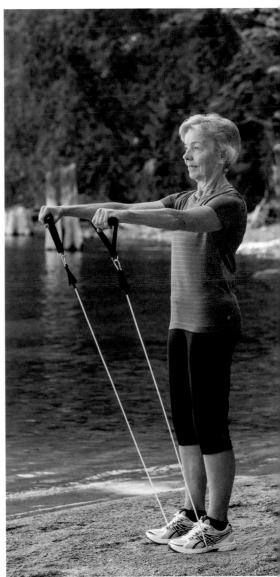

HIGH CURL

This curl variation works your biceps from an angle unique to resistance bands and cable machines at the gym; this angle wouldn't be possible using dumbbells or barbells.

Stand in front of your anchor point, set to shoulder height. Hold a resistance band handle in each hand, with your palms facing up.

Keep your upper arms stable as you bring your hands toward your head. Only your forearms should move (not your upper arms). Pause briefly, then straighten your arms to return to the start position.

Avoid the tendency to curl your wrists toward you as you bring the resistance band handles toward your head; keep them in line with your forearms.

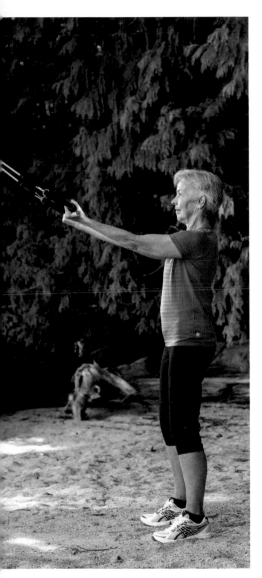

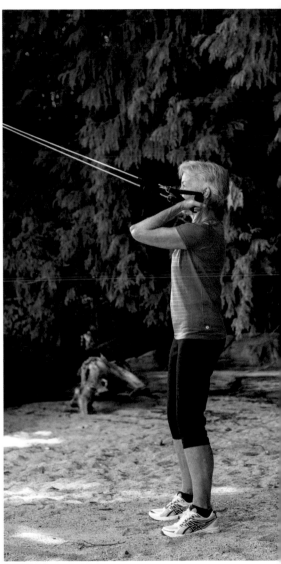

INCLINE CHEST PRESS

Compared to the "regular" chest press, this variation puts a bit more emphasis on the shoulders. It also works the pectorals (chest muscles) and triceps.

Stand facing away from your anchor point, set to about ankle height. Start with each side of the band under your arms, with your hands to the sides of your chest. You can stand with your feet hip width apart and knees slightly bent, or in a split stance with one foot in front of the other (I find the latter option more stable when using heavier resistance).

Press the resistance band handles out and up, bringing your hands closer together (but not touching) near the end of the movement. Your hands will come to about eye level. This mimics an incline dumbbell bench press movement, in which you'd start with dumbbells on either side of your chest, bringing them to almost touching as you extend your arms.

Bring your hands back to the start position, and repeat for reps.

As you start using heavier resistance levels, you may find that you need to lean forward slightly so you're not pulled backward. This is perfectly fine—just make sure that your torso stays in the same position throughout each set, rather than leaning backwards and forwards with each rep.

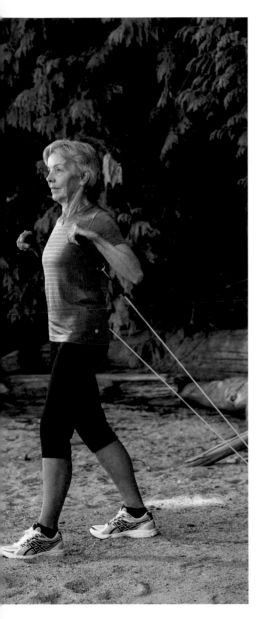
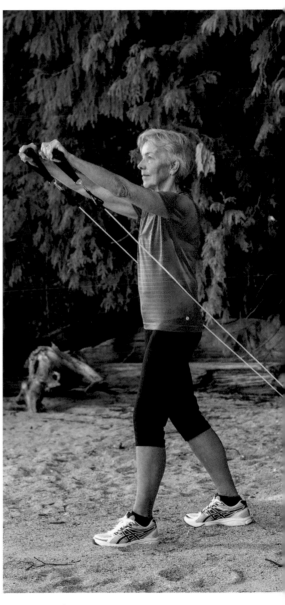

INCLINE PUSH-UP

The push-up is a fundamental upper body strength movement that works your chest, shoulders, triceps, and core. Adding a mini-band around your wrists adds a unique challenge, and can help to keep your upper arms and elbows in the correct position.

Start with a higher incline, such as a countertop. When you feel comfortable performing 10 reps in a row with good form, progress to a slightly lower incline. Our model here is using a challengingly low incline!

Loop a mini-band around your wrists. Start in a plank position on your hands and toes, with your wrists just in front of your shoulders and your hands shoulder-width apart and elevated on a stable surface. Brace your abs and squeeze your glutes, making sure your head, torso, hips, and legs are in line.

Maintaining your plank position, bend your arms to bring your chest toward your hands. When your chest comes to within a few inches of your hands, straighten your arms and press back up into the start position. Maintain tension on the mini-band throughout the movement. Think of a push-up as a moving plank: your body moves as one unit.

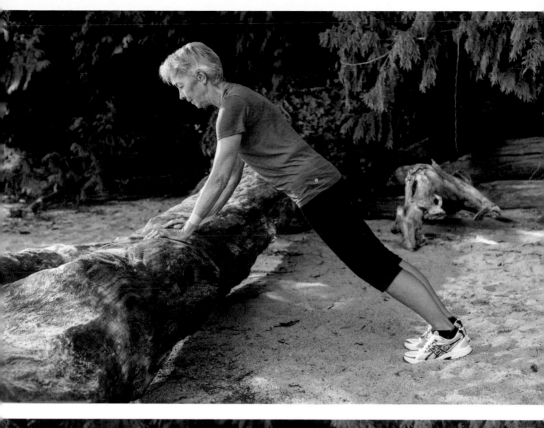
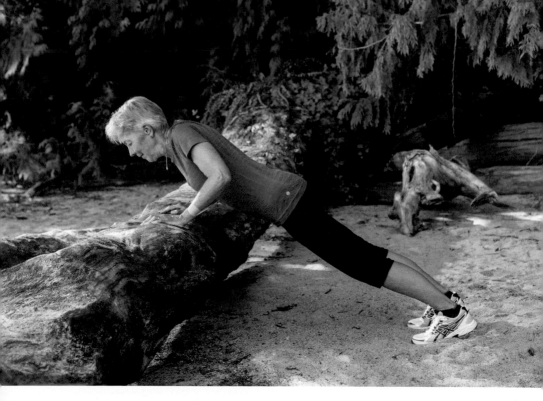

KNEELING PULL-DOWN

This move targets the major muscles in your back—especially the latissimus dorsi—and can help improve your posture.

Anchor your resistance band above head height. Get into a half-kneeling position, facing the anchor point. One leg should be bent in front of you, with the other knee on the ground directly below your hip.

Start with your arms straight and reaching up at about a 45-degree angle, palms facing away from you. Make sure your shoulders are down and away from your ears. Row the band handles to your shoulders, keeping your palms facing forward throughout, and squeezing your shoulder blades together as you perform this movement. Hold the contracted position for a second, then straighten your arms to return to the start position.

For back-strengthening movements like this one, try holding the resistance band handles with a loose grip, focusing on using your back muscles to pull the band, rather than your hands.

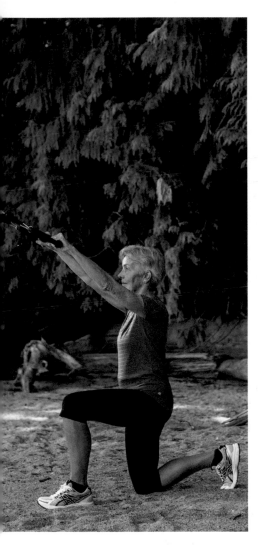
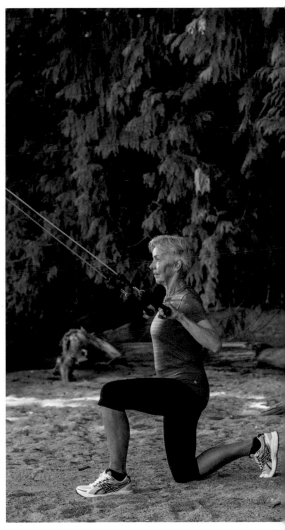

LATERAL RAISE

This exercise focuses on the lateral head of the deltoid (shoulder) muscle. For the best shoulder health and muscle development, make sure you round out your shoulder training by including moves to target the other muscle heads as well, such as rear delt flys and front raises.

Stand with both feet on a resistance band, hands at your sides and knees slightly bent. Make sure your shoulders are down and away from your ears, and your shoulder blades are lightly squeezed together.

Keeping your arms straight, raise your arms until they're a little higher than parallel to the floor. Hold the contracted position for a second, then lower back to the start position.

Make sure you maintain perfect posture throughout the movement, with your head in line with your spine, and back neutral (not hyperextended). Avoid the tendency to lean back as you raise your arms, especially with heavier resistance levels.

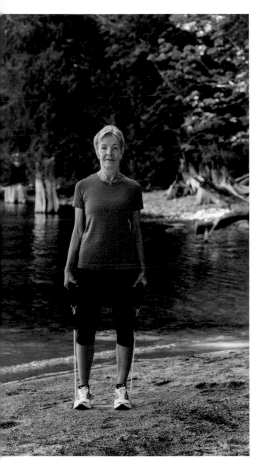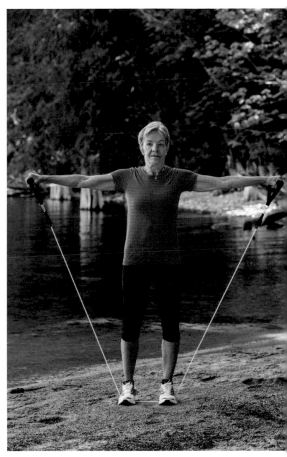

LOW CURL

This biceps curl variation is unique to resistance bands (and gym cable machines); this angle of resistance would be impossible to achieve using dumbbells or a barbell.

Stand facing away from your anchor point, set to ankle height. Hold a resistance band handle in each hand, palms facing up, with your hands slightly behind your thighs. Make sure you feel resistance from the band in this position.

Keep your upper arms stable as you bring your hands toward your shoulders. Only your forearms should move (not your upper arms). Pause briefly, then straighten your arms to return to the start position.

Avoid the tendency to curl your wrists toward you as you bring the resistance band handles toward your shoulders; keep them in line with your forearms throughout the movement.

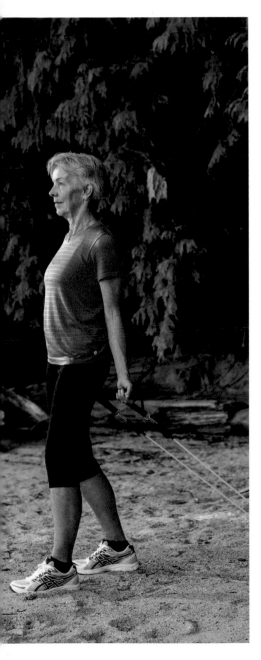
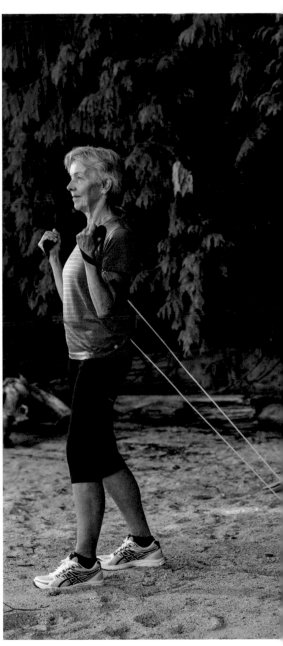

OVERHEAD EXTENSION

This movement targets the triceps, the largest muscle group in our arms.

Stand facing away from your anchor point, set to just above head height. Hold a resistance band handle in each hand behind your head. Place one foot in front of the other, and lean forward slightly. Make sure your spine stays in a neutral position; avoid rounding or hyperextending your back.

Keeping your elbows close to your head, start with your elbows bent, and hands reaching towards your back. You should feel tension on the resistance band in this starting position, as well as a stretch in your triceps.

Straighten your arms, bringing your hands overhead. Once your elbows straighten, flex your triceps and hold the contracted position for a second, then return to the start position.

Make sure your upper arms stay in place throughout the movement, and your elbows don't flare out to each side of your head.

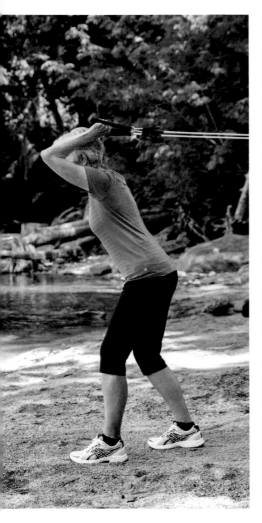
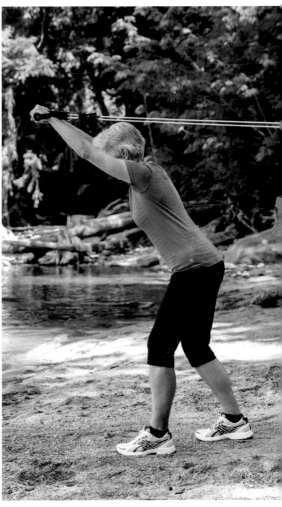

OVERHEAD PRESS

The overhead press is one of the most important and effective shoulder strength movements. Other than increasing strength in the shoulders, it activates the entire core musculature, and can help develop a strong bench press if you lift weights in a gym.

Stand with both feet on a resistance band, hip width apart. Hold the handles in front of your shoulders, with your palms facing away from you. Brace your abdominal muscles (as if you were about to cough) and squeeze your glutes.

Maintaining this posture, press the band handles overhead, moving your hands slightly closer together near the top of the move. Your arms should be straight, and your biceps should be next to your ears. Reverse the movement to return to the start position.

Make sure you keep your glutes and abs activated throughout this movement to prevent hyperextending your spine, especially when you're using a challenging resistance level.

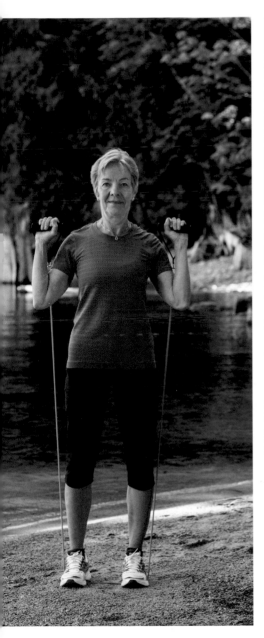
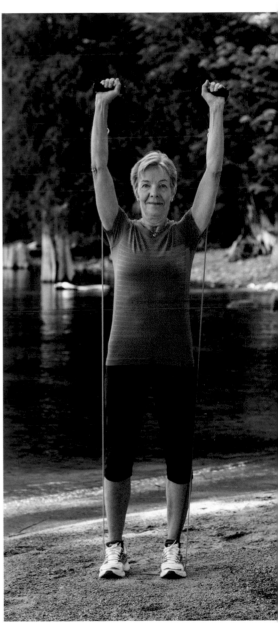

PEC FLY

In addition to strengthening the pectoral (chest) muscles, this move can help improve posture by stretching out the chest muscles and helping you squeeze your shoulder blades together in the start position of the exercise.

Stand facing away from your anchor point, set to about chest height. Place one foot in front of the other, and lean forward slightly. Make sure your spine stays in a neutral position; avoid rounding or hyperextending your back.

Start with your arms mostly straight—just a slight bend in your elbows—with your hands just behind your back. You should feel a slight stretch in your chest muscles.

Without changing the angle of your elbows, and keeping your arms parallel to the ground, bring the resistance band handles together in front of your chest until your hands touch.

Hold the contraction briefly, then slowly reach your arms back to the start position.

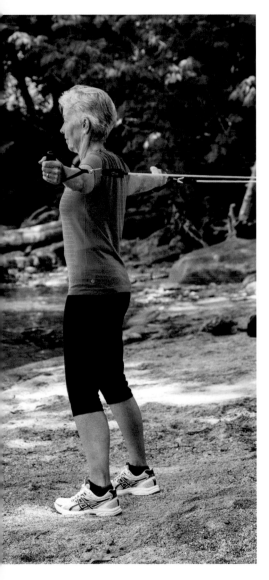
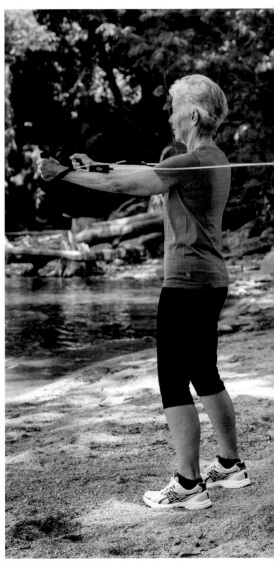

STANDING REAR DELT FLY

This exercise strengthens the posterior deltoid (a.k.a. rear delt), the back portion of the shoulder muscle. It's a relatively small muscle, so this move doesn't require a lot of resistance compared to other moves. The rear delts are extremely important to maintaining good posture and overall shoulder health.

Stand facing your anchor point, set to about eye level, with your feet hip width apart. Start with your arms straight out in front of you at shoulder height, palms facing each other.

Keeping your shoulders down and away from your ears and keeping your arms straight (or a very slight bend in your elbows if that's more comfortable), bring your arms out to your sides until your hands are just past your back. Pause briefly, then return to the start position and repeat for reps.

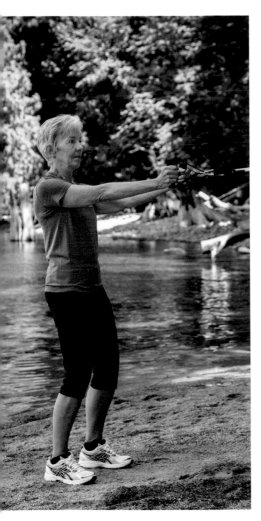
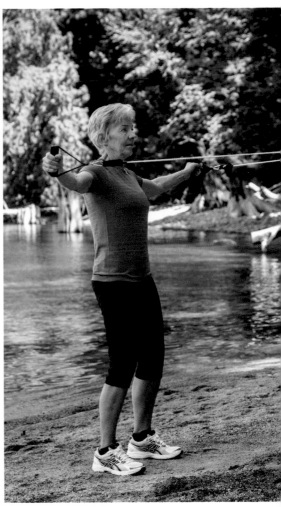

STANDING ROW

Rows are one of the most effective movements you can perform to improve your posture and strengthen the muscles of your back, including the rhomboids and latissimus dorsi. You'll also work your biceps, forearms, and shoulders.

Stand facing your anchor point, set to about chest height, with your feet hip width apart, knees bent slightly, and a neutral spine (head not poking forward, back flat).

Start with your arms straight out in front of you, palms facing each other. Make sure your shoulders are down and away from your ears.

Row the band handles toward your chest, squeezing your shoulder blades together as your arms move. Hold the contracted position for a second, then straighten your arms to return to the start position.

As you start using heavier resistance levels, you may find that you need to lean backward slightly and bend your knees so you're not pulled forward. This is perfectly fine; just make sure that your torso stays in the same position throughout each set, rather than leaning backwards and forwards with each rep.

For back-strengthening movements like this one, try holding the resistance band handles with a loose grip, focusing on using your back muscles to pull the band, rather than your hands.

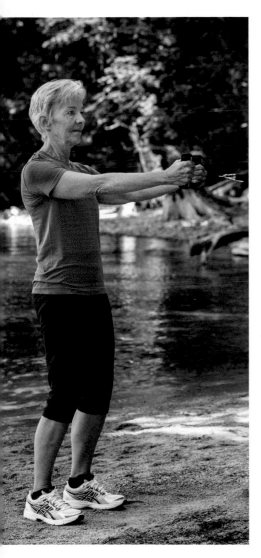
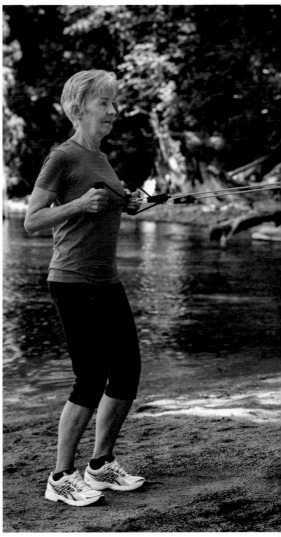

STANDING WIDE ROW

This row variation focuses on the latissimus dorsi muscle, the largest muscle in the back. You'll also work your biceps, forearms, and shoulders.

Stand facing your anchor point, set to about chest height, with your feet hip width apart, knees bent slightly, and a neutral spine (head not poking forward, back flat).

Start with your arms straight out in front of you, palms facing the ground. Make sure your shoulders are down and away from your ears.

Row the band handles out to each side of your chest, squeezing your shoulder blades together as your arms move. Your elbows should be bent at approximately 90 degrees, with your forearms pointing straight forward. Hold the contracted position for a second, then straighten your arms to return to the start position.

As you start using heavier resistance levels, you may find that you need to lean backward slightly and bend your knees so you're not pulled forward. This is perfectly fine; just make sure that your torso stays in the same position throughout each set, rather than leaning backwards and forwards with each rep.

For back-strengthening movements like this one, try holding the resistance band handles with a loose grip, focusing on using your back muscles to pull the band, rather than your hands.

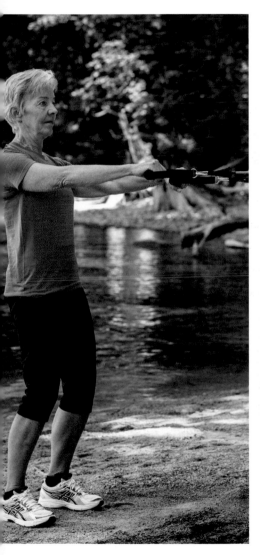
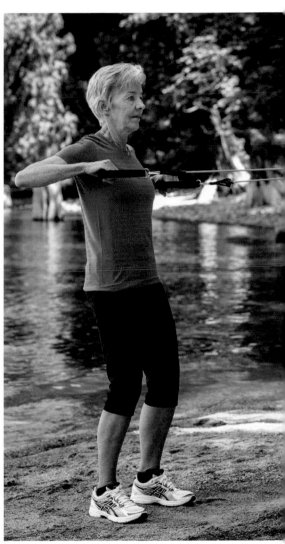

STRAIGHT ARM PULLDOWN

This exercise targets the latissiumus dorsi (called "lats" for short), the muscles along the sides of your back. It's great for people who find it difficult to feel the lats engaging in other pulldown variations.

Anchor your resistance band just above head height. Face the anchor point and stand with your feet hip width apart. Hinge your hips back, bending your knees until your torso is at a 30- to 45-degree angle. Extend your arms in front of you, making sure you feel some tension on the resistance band.

Keeping your elbows straight, press your arms to your sides, bringing your hands in line with your hips, or slightly behind them.

Make sure you keep your elbows straight. Bending your arms will engage the triceps instead of the lats.

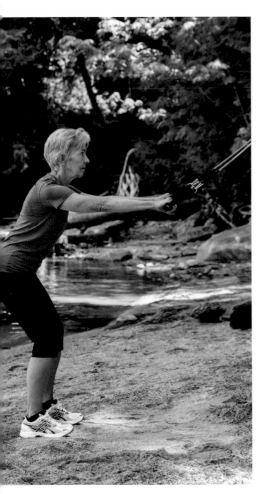
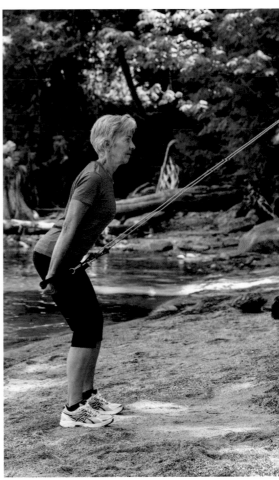

SUPERBAND SEATED ROW

This row variation mimics a cable seated row you might perform at the gym. It's a very effective exercise for all your postural muscles, including your rhomboids and lats. You don't need an anchor point for a band (you provide your own!), and this exercise may be more comfortable than bent-over rows for those with low back pain.

Sit on the ground with your legs in front of you and your feet together. You can have your legs straight or your knees slightly bent—whichever is more comfortable.

Loop a superband around your feet, and hold one side in each hand just above your knees. Start with your arms straight, chest tall, and a slight backward lean with your torso.

Keeping your shoulders down and away from your ears, row the band toward your midsection, focusing on squeezing your shoulder blades together as you row. Hold the contraction briefly, then return to the start position.

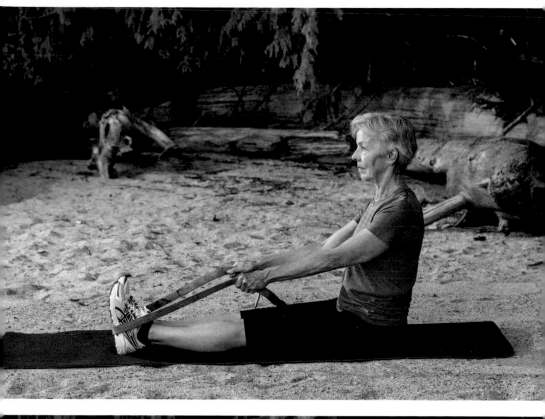

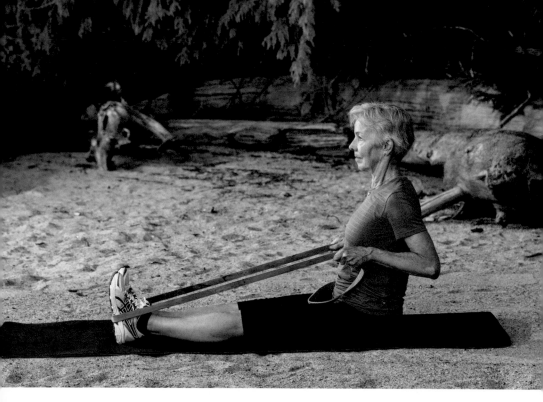

TRICEPS KICKBACK

This isolation exercise for the triceps builds strength and muscle on the back of your arms.

Anchor your resistance band at about chest height. Stand facing the anchor point, holding one end of the band in each hand (you may find this more comfortable than holding the handles).

Hinge your hips back behind you and bend your torso forward, keeping your spine neutral and your head in line with your spine. You should have your knees slightly bent, with most of your weight on your heels. Start with your elbows pinned to your sides, palms facing each other, and shoulder blades squeezed together.

Without moving your upper arms, extend your forearms so your elbows are straight. Hold this contracted position for a second, then return to the start position.

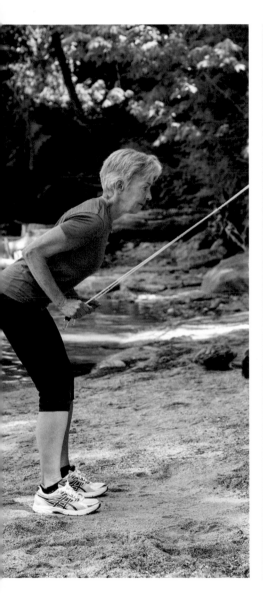 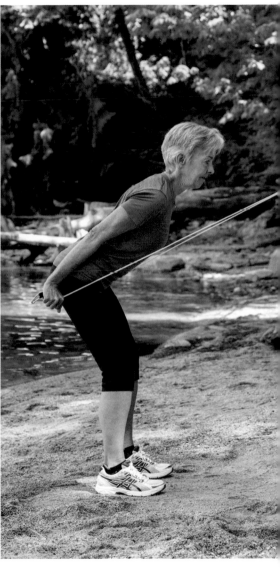

TRICEPS PRESS-DOWN

The triceps are the largest muscles of the arm. Strong triceps help you perform pushing movements like chest presses and push-ups.

Stand facing your anchor point, set to above head height, with a resistance band handle in each hand and palms facing up. Pin your elbows to your sides, keep your shoulders down and away from your ears, and squeeze your shoulder blades together. Start with your hands in front of your chest.

Keeping your upper arms stable, press your hands down until your arms are straight. Pause briefly, then return to the start position.

Avoid the tendency to curl your wrists toward you; keep them in line with your forearms.

You can also try this move with your palms facing down; many people find this slightly easier.

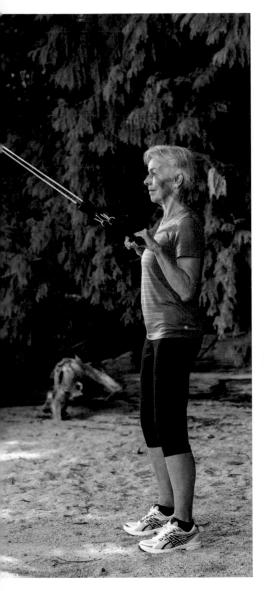
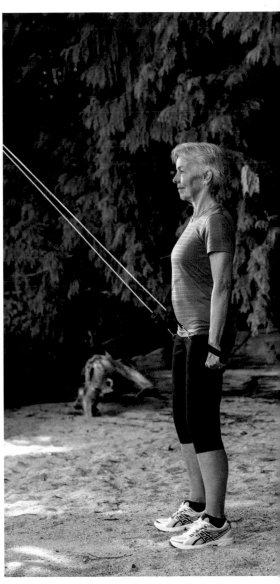

LOWER BODY EXERCISES

BANDED SQUAT

Squats are one of the most important lower body strength movements. Using a mini-band above your knees is a great way to practice good squat form; one of the most common form faults when people perform squats is having the knees cave in toward each other. Pressing your knees against the tension of your mini-band will prevent this!

Stand with a mini-band looped just above your knees, with your feet hip width or slightly further apart. Your toes can be pointed forward or angled out slightly. Keep your hands at chest level, elbows bent.

Keeping your knees in line with your toes (working against the tension of the band to ensure your knees don't cave inward), bend your knees and flex your hips until your thighs are parallel to the ground, and your knees are bent at 90 degrees. Make sure your spine stays in a neutral position throughout the movement, and your weight is evenly distributed along each foot.

Press through your feet to return to standing, squeezing your glutes as you ascend.

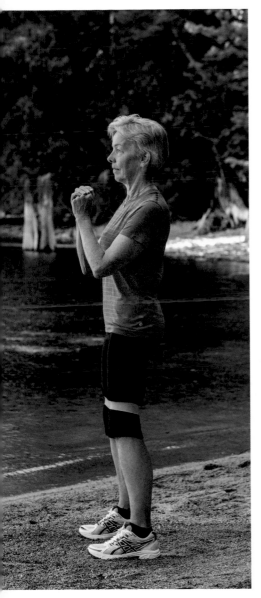
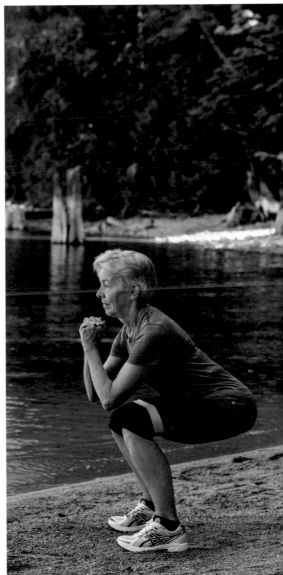

CLAMSHELL

This movement focuses on the gluteus medius muscles (the sides of your glutes), which stabilize the pelvis during single leg stances. The gluteus medius also externally rotates the hip, which is what happens in this clamshell exercise.

Place a mini-band above your knees. Lie on the floor on your left side, supporting your head with your left hand, elbow on the floor. Bend your knees to about 90 degrees.

Keep your core braced as you rotate your right hip, moving your right knee away from your left knee. With the resistance of the band, you should feel your outer right glute working. Move as far as you can without initiating movement anywhere other than your right leg (such as hyperextending your low back). Pause for a second, then smoothly return your right leg to the start position. Perform all reps on one side, then switch sides.

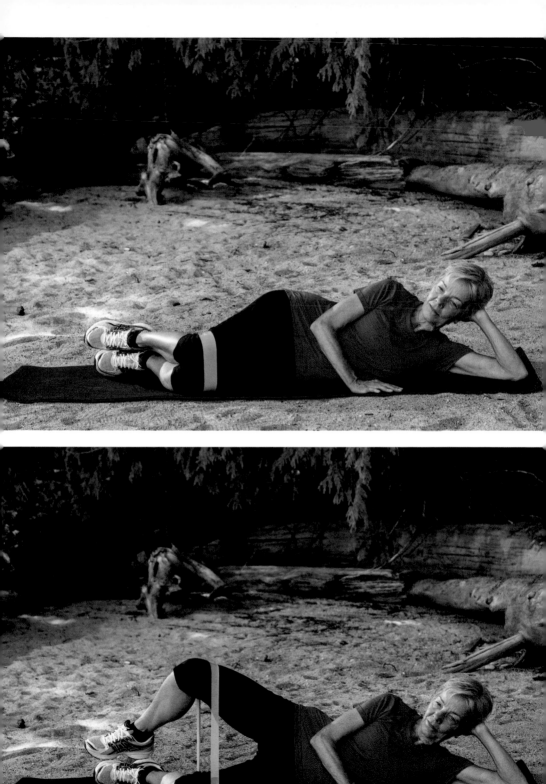

GLUTE BRIDGE

This exercise targets the largest muscle group in the human body: the glutes. Strengthening your glutes can alleviate and prevent low back and knee pain.

Lie on your back with a mini-band looped just above your knees. Place your feet hip width apart, with your heels close to your glutes. Keep each knee in line with each mid-foot; you should feel your outer glutes (gluteus medius) working against the tension of the band.

Tuck your pelvis so there's no space between your low back and the floor. Maintain this back position throughout the exercise.

Press through your heels as you raise your hips off the floor, squeezing your glutes. Your body should form a straight line from your chest to your knees, and your shins should be perpendicular to the floor. Hold this position briefly, then return to the start position.

Variation: To make this move extra challenging, at the top of the move, add abduction: move your knees farther apart from each other, as far as you can go while maintaining body alignment. Bring them back to neutral (each knee above each foot) before lowering back to the start position.

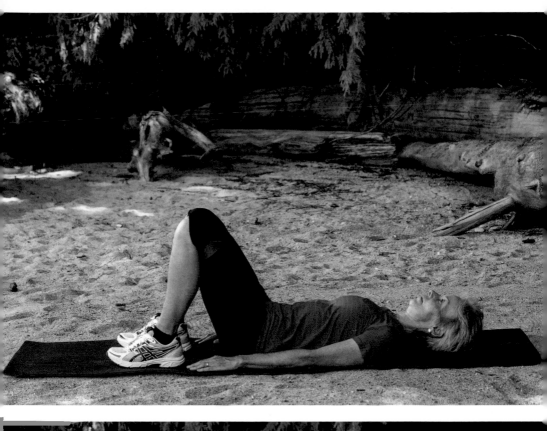
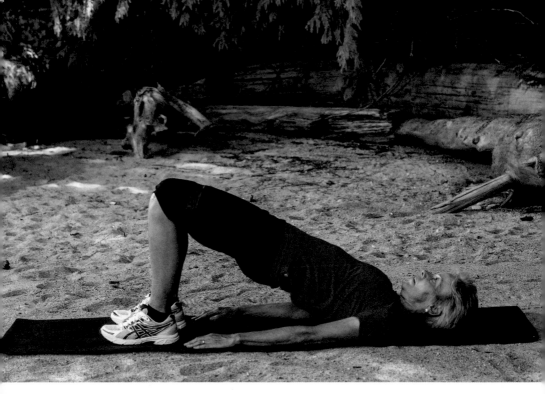

SUPERBAND HIP HINGE

This resistance band hip hinge variation is an excellent way to practice good deadlift form. Having the resistance band pull your hips backward "grooves" the movement pattern of a hip hinge, ensuring you're using the correct muscles to perform the exercise.

Anchor a pull-up assistance band at about ankle height. Stand facing away from the anchor point, with the band around your hips and your arms straight out in front of you.

Hinge your hips back behind you, making sure you feel most of the work in your hamstrings and glutes. Keep your spine neutral, and your head in line with your spine. In this bottom position, you should be looking at the ground about three feet in front of you. Make sure you feel tension on the band in this position.

Using your hamstrings and glutes, thrust your hips forward to come to standing. Squeeze your glutes at the top position, then repeat for reps.

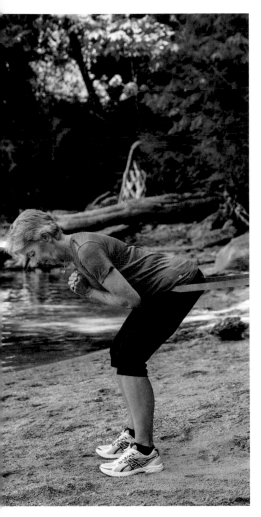

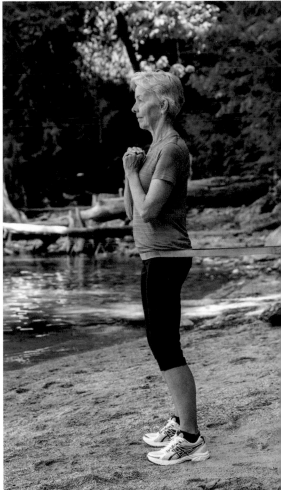

KICKSTAND DEADLIFT

Unilateral movements (which work one side at a time) like this one are very important to preventing injury and improving athletic performance. Most of us have a dominant, and thus stronger, side. Working each side separately can balance out differences between sides. The kickstand deadlift strengthens your hamstrings and glutes, while improving your balance.

Stand upright with your left foot on the middle of a resistance band. Hold a resistance band handle in each hand, arms straight, with your hands in front of your thighs. To create enough tension for this exercise, you'll likely need to coil or fold the band a few times, and place that under your foot. Most of your weight should be on your left leg, with your right foot lightly touching the ground just behind your left foot.

Hinging your hips back behind you, bend your left knee slightly as you lean your torso forward. Keeping the ball of your right foot lightly touching the ground and keeping your arms straight throughout the movement, bring your hands a few inches past your knee. Keep your head in line with your spine; in this bottom position, you should be looking at the ground a few feet in front of you, rather than straight ahead.

Press through your left heel to return to the start position. Keep your spine neutral for the duration of the exercise.

Complete all reps on one side, then switch sides.

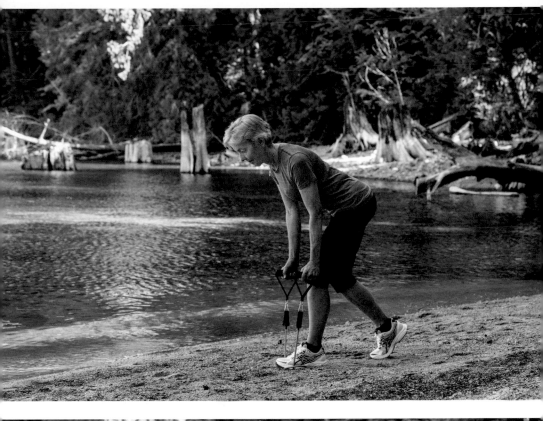

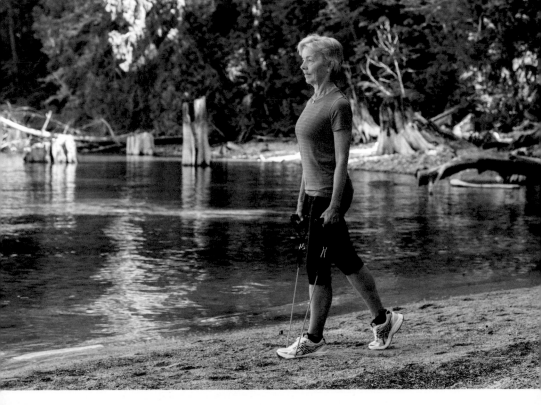

LATERAL WALK

This exercise targets the gluteus medius muscles (the sides of your glutes). It's an excellent movement to perform as a warm-up before engaging in a lower-body-intensive workout.

With a mini-band looped above your knees, stand with your hands on your hips, feet hip width apart, and your knees slightly bent. Keeping your knees in line with your tocs (don't let your knees fall inwards), take a step to the left with your left foot. Follow with a step to the left with your right foot, placing it under your right hip.

Make sure you don't drag your trailing foot on the ground; take deliberate steps. Also make sure you keep your torso perfectly upright, without leaning to the side. Throughout the exercise, your head, torso, and hips should remain in a stacked position.

Complete all your reps moving to the left, then switch directions.

You should feel this move primarily in your glutes. To increase the challenge level, loop a mini-band around your ankles instead of above your knees. If one mini-band isn't challenging enough, use one around your ankles, and a second above your knees.

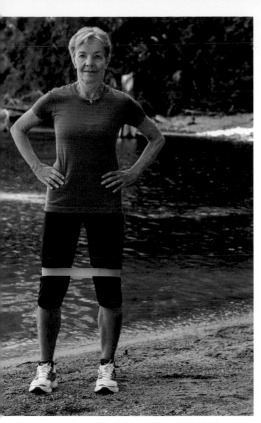
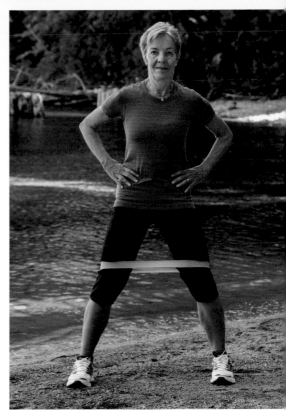
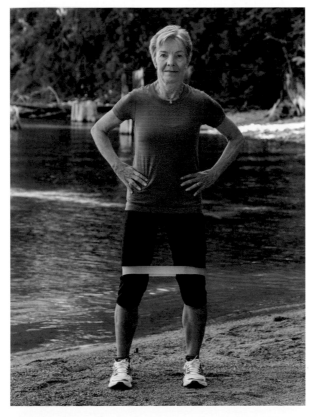

LYING ABDUCTION

This exercise strengthens the gluteus medius muscle, on the side of your hips. It's extremely important for maintaining good form while running or walking, as it stabilizes your pelvis while one leg is off the ground.

Lie on the ground on your left side, supporting your head with your left hand. Place your right hand on the ground in front of you, or on your right hip.

With a mini-band looped around your ankles, straighten your legs and stack your feet on top of each other.

Raise your right leg until it forms a 45-degree angle with the ground. Pause briefly, then return to the start position and repeat for reps before switching to the other side.

Keep your right foot flexed throughout the movement, with your toes pointing forward (not upwards).

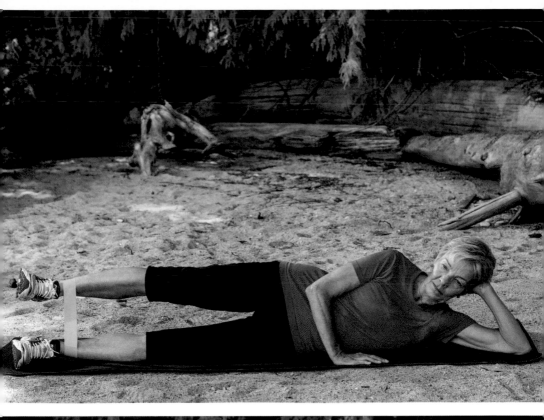

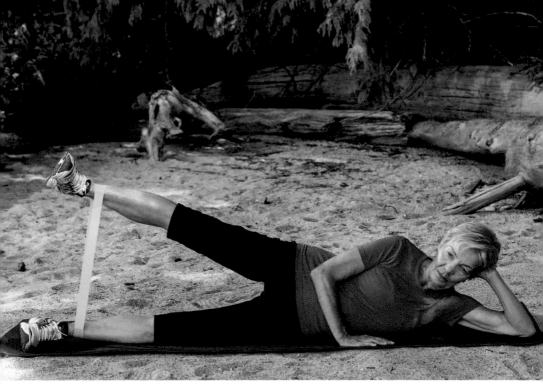

PULL-THROUGH

This hip hinge movement focuses on the hamstrings and glutes, and is an excellent exercise for practicing deadlift form.

Set your resistance band anchor point to about ankle height. Facing away from the anchor and holding a resistance band handle in each hand, stand with your feet hip width apart. Hinge your hips backward toward the anchor point, bending your knees and keeping your spine neutral. You should feel your hamstrings activating, and you should have most of your weight on your heels. Keep your head in line with your spine; in this bottom position, you should be looking at the ground a few feet in front of you, rather than looking straight ahead.

Keeping your hands between your legs, thrust your hips forward, squeezing your glutes. You should be fully upright in this ending position, with your head, shoulders, hips, knees, and ankles in line. Hold the contraction briefly, then hinge your hips back to return to the start position.

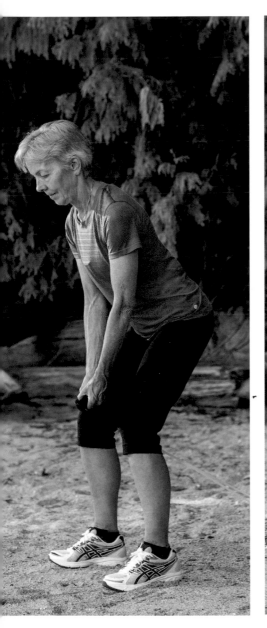
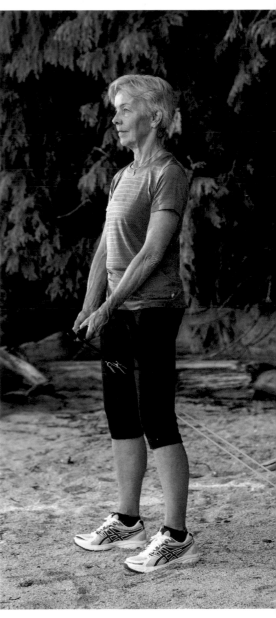

QUADRUPED KICKBACK

This move strengthens the glutes, while also working the entire musculature of the core.

Holding a resistance band handle in each hand, get onto all fours on the floor. Loop the resistance band around the middle of your left foot. Start with your hands directly under your shoulders, and your knees under your hips. Brace your abs.

Keeping your hips and shoulders stable, squeeze your left glute as you extend your left leg. Bring it parallel to the floor and make sure it's completely straight. Hold this contracted position briefly, then return to the start position.

Make sure you don't bring your leg much higher than parallel to the floor, as you'll hyperextend your low back. Perform all reps on one side, then switch sides.

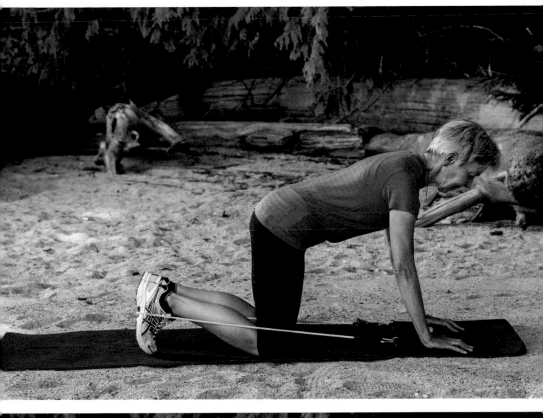
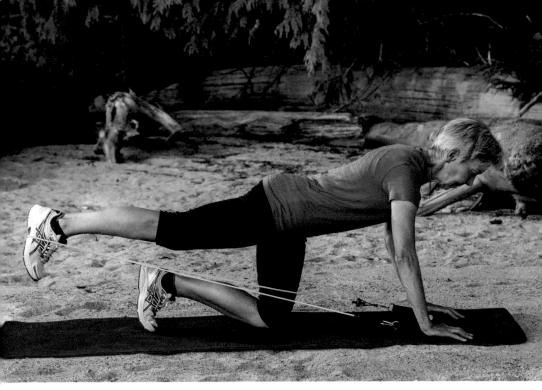

SIDE LUNGE

This unique lunge variation works both your core and your lower body. As an anti-rotational core movement, you'll be using your obliques to keep your hands centered in front of your chest; tension from the band will be pulling your arms to one side.

Holding both resistance band handles together in both hands, stand to the right of your anchor point, set to about chest height. With your arms straight, position your hands in the center of your chest, and ensure you have some tension on the band.

Take a large step out to your right side, keeping your left leg straight and bending your right knee as far as you comfortably can. See if you can feel a stretch in your left adductor (inner thigh) muscle. Try to keep your torso as upright as possible. A bit of forward lean—as long as your back is flat—is fine. Your goal is to keep your hands in the center of your chest throughout the movement.

Push off your right foot to return to the start position. Repeat for reps, then switch to the other side.

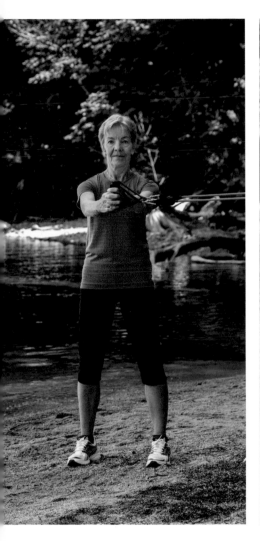
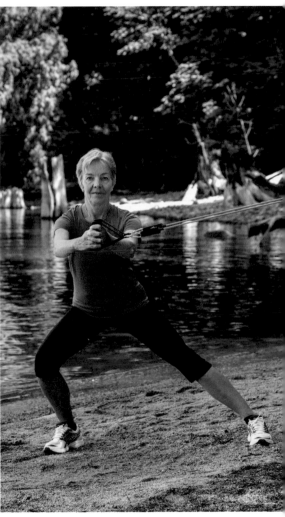

SINGLE LEG GLUTE BRIDGE

This is a more challenging variation of the regular glute bridge. Since you're working one leg at a time, this exercise can help even out any strength imbalances between the left and right sides.

Lie on your back with a mini-band looped just above your knees. Place your feet hip width apart, with your heels close to your glutes. Lift your right foot off the ground and point your leg toward the ceiling (your leg doesn't need to be perfectly straight). Keep your left knee in line with your left mid-foot, and make sure your right thigh stays parallel to your left, rather than getting pulled inward by the band. You should feel your outer glutes (gluteus medius) working against the tension of the band.

Tuck your pelvis so there's no space between your low back and the floor. Maintain this back position throughout the exercise.

Press through your left heel as you raise your hips off the floor, squeezing your glutes. Your body should form a straight line from your chest to your left knee, and your left shin should be perpendicular to the floor. Hold this position briefly, then return to the start position.

Perform all reps on one side, then switch sides.

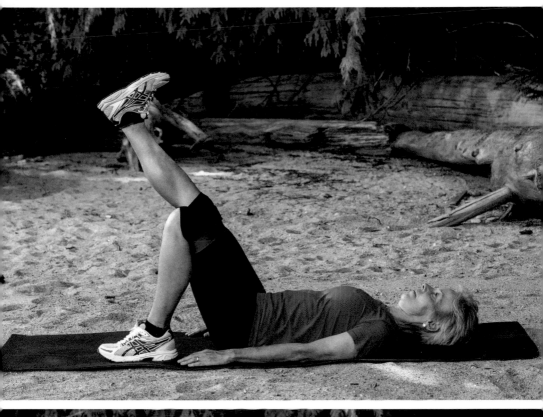

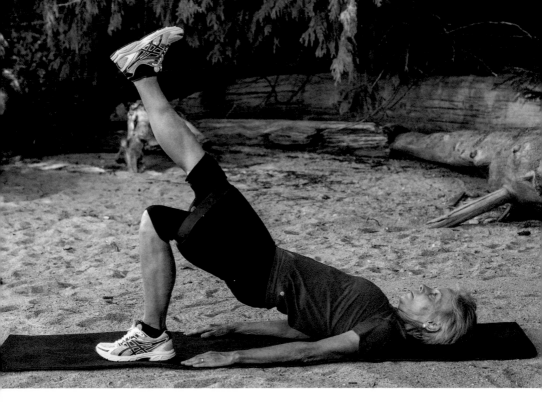

SINGLE LEG HIP EXTENSION

This move isolates the glutes. Strong glutes are extremely important for preventing low back pain, preventing injury, and increasing athletic performance.

Set up a resistance band in an anchor set to about ankle height. If your resistance band set came with an ankle strap, use that for this movement. If not, you can place your foot into one of the regular handles.

Face the anchor point and start with the strap around your left ankle (or handle around your left foot). Keeping your back straight and right knee slightly bent, you can place one or both hands on the wall in front of you for support, if needed.

Extend your left leg behind you, squeezing your left glute and keeping your left leg straight. Pause at the top of the movement, then slowly bring your leg back to the start position.

Make sure you don't lift your working leg too high; you'll hyperextend your low back. You should feel this move in both of your glutes. Your left glute is working against the resistance of the band, and your right glute is stabilizing you.

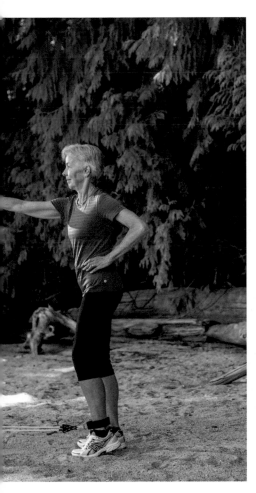
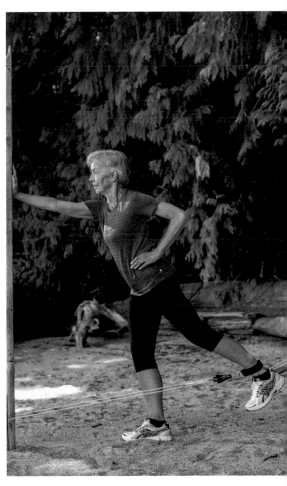

SPLIT SQUAT

Split squats work all the major muscles of the lower body, including the glutes, quads, and hamstrings.

Stand with your left foot in the middle of a resistance band, holding a handle in each hand at shoulder height. Step back with your right foot and balance on the ball of your foot. Keep your back straight and your head in line with your spine.

Keeping the resistance band handles at shoulder height, bend both knees until your left thigh is parallel to the ground. Both knees should be bent at 90 degrees, and your right knee should be just above the ground.

Press through your left foot to straighten your legs and return to the start position. Throughout the exercise, make sure that your head, torso, and hips remain in a stacked position.

Perform all reps on one side, then switch sides.

This move can also be performed as a reverse lunge: instead of keeping your feet in the same position throughout each set, you can step one foot behind you, lower into a lunge, and step that foot back to the start position with each rep.

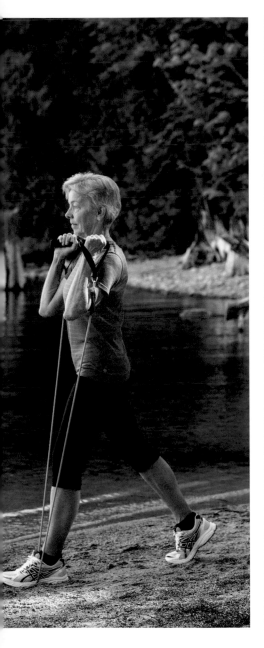

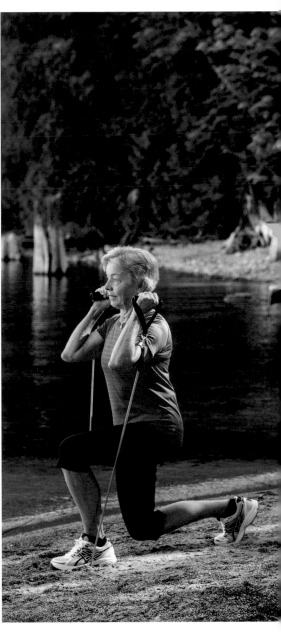

SUPERBAND DEADLIFT

This unique deadlift variation works your hamstrings, glutes, and spinal erector muscles.

With your feet hip width apart, loop a superband around each mid-foot. Grab the middle of the superband with both hands.

Hinge your hips back behind you, making sure you feel most of the work in your hamstrings and glutes. Keep your spine neutral, and your head in line with your spine. In this bottom position, you should be looking at the ground about three feet in front of you.

Using your hamstrings and glutes, thrust your hips forward to come to standing. Squeeze your glutes at the top position, then repeat for reps.

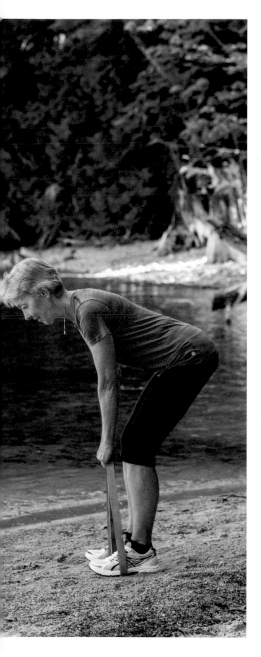
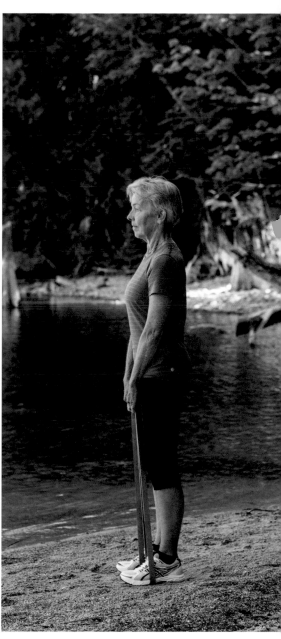

SUPERBAND SINGLE LEG PRESS

This exercise mimics the leg press machine, where you push a loaded platform away from you with your leg muscles. Here, you're creating load by anchoring a superband in your hands.

Lie on your back, with your left leg extended straight along the ground, and a superband looped around your right foot. Start with your right thigh perpendicular to the ground, and your knee bent at 90 degrees. Hold the superband at either side of your right thigh.

Keeping your hands in place, press your right foot against the band, straightening your leg. It should create a 45-degree angle with the floor. Hold the contraction briefly, then reverse the motion and return to the start position.

Repeat all reps on one side, then switch sides.

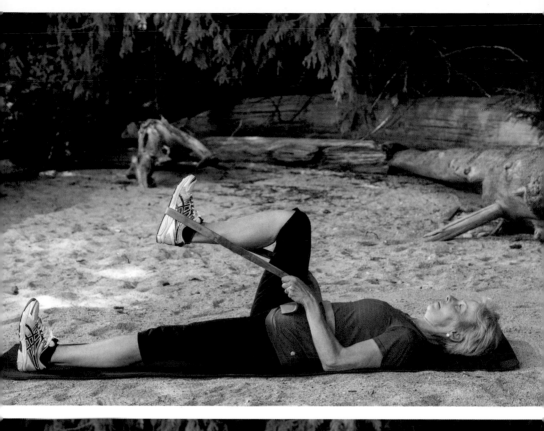

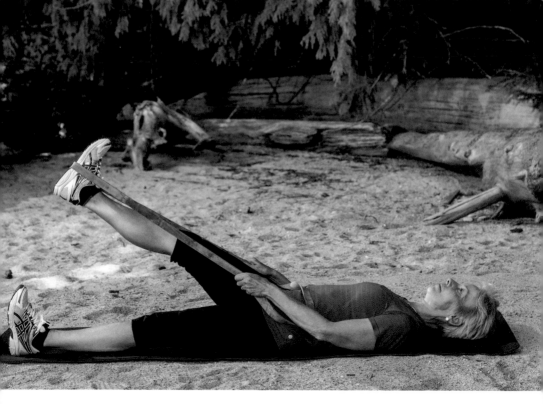

SUPERBAND SIDE LUNGE

Side lunges develop balance and stability in addition to strength. In this side lunge variation, you'll focus on your quads, hamstrings, and glutes (the resistance band version on page 100 also works your core).

Stand to the right of your anchor point, set to about hip height. Loop a superband around your hips, and ensure you have some tension on the band.

Take a large step out to your right side, keeping your left leg straight and bending your right knee as far as you comfortably can. See if you can feel a stretch in your left adductor (inner thigh) muscle. Try to keep your torso as upright as possible. A bit of forward lean—as long as your back is flat—is fine.

Push off your right foot to return to the start position. Repeat for reps, then switch to the other side.

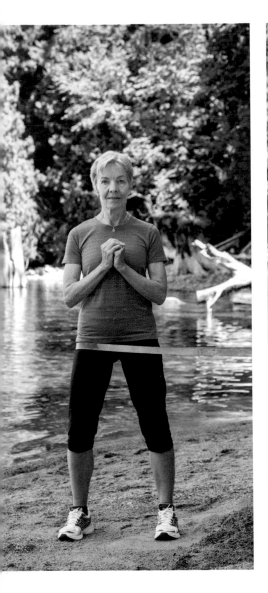
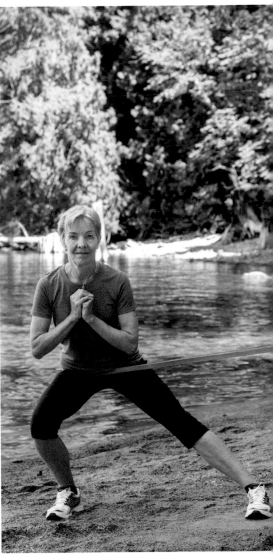

TORSO ROTATION

Targeting your transverse abdominis and oblique muscles, this exercise involves more rotational movement than the high-low and low-high chops.

Stand with your feet hip width apart, to the right of a resistance band anchored at about chest height. Hold both resistance handles together. Start with your arms straight and extended to your left, knees slightly bent.

Using your oblique muscles to initiate the movement, move the band handles in a smooth arc to your right, keeping your arms at chest height throughout the movement.

Make sure you're initiating this movement with your abs (specifically your obliques), not your arms. It should feel like your arms are just going along for the ride!

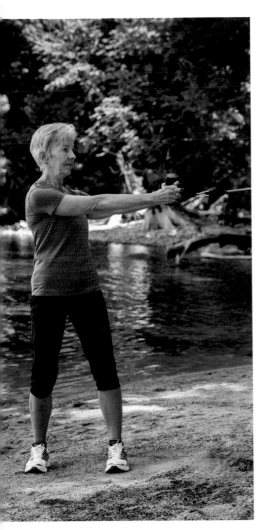
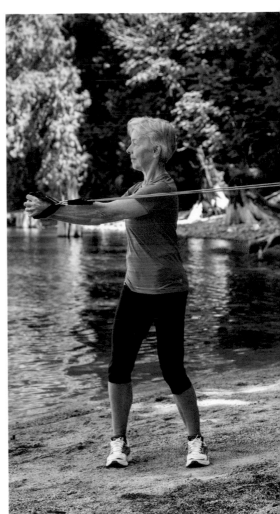

CORE EXERCISES

BICYCLE CRUNCH

Adding a mini-band to this classic core exercise strengthens the hip flexor muscles, and also helps you maintain correct form. If you don't keep your extended leg engaged, the band will go slack!

Lie on the floor with your hands behind your head and legs bent at 90 degrees (feet off the floor). Loop a mini-band around the middle of your feet. Make sure you're not pulling your head forward; your hands should lightly support your head.

Brace your abs and raise your upper back off the floor. Aim your right shoulder toward your left hip as you straighten your left leg. Pull your right knee toward your chest as you bring your left leg toward the ground. Lower your leg as far as you can while keeping your low back in contact with the floor.

Maintain tension on the mini-band as you reverse the motion, bending your left knee and bringing it toward your chest as you straighten your right leg toward the floor, rotating your torso to the left.

You can also perform this move by twisting toward each bent leg, rather than twisting toward the straight leg. Try it both ways!

This exercise is often performed too quickly. To ensure you're not using momentum and are effectively training your abs, it should take 2 to 3 seconds to lower each leg toward the floor. For this exercise, alternate sides with each rep.

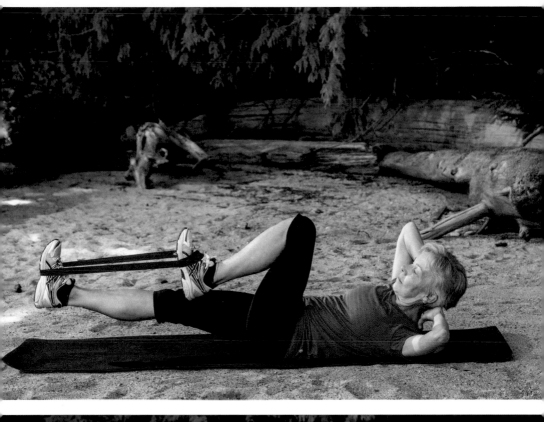

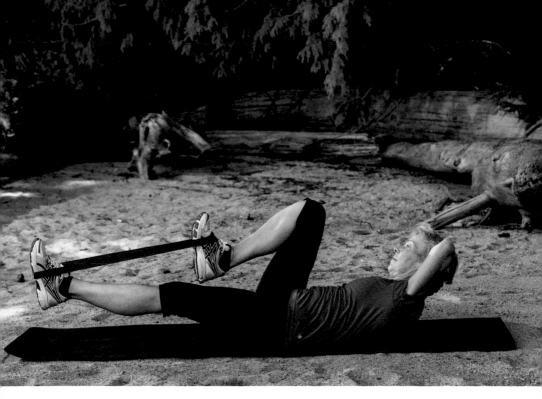

HIGH-LOW CHOP

Chops target the transverse abdominis and oblique muscles in your core, while strengthening the rotational movement pattern. This is beneficial for any twisting motion like throwing, boxing, or golfing.

Stand with your feet hip width apart, to the right of a resistance band anchored just above head height. Hold both resistance band handles together. Start with your arms straight and extended to your left, hands at head height, knees slightly bent.

Using your core muscles to initiate the movement, move the band handles in a smooth arc to your right, ending with your hands at about hip height. Perform all reps on one side, then switch sides.

Make sure you're initiating this movement with your abs (specifically your obliques), not your arms. It should feel like your arms are just going along for the ride!

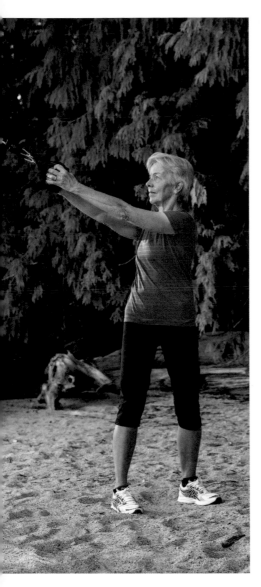
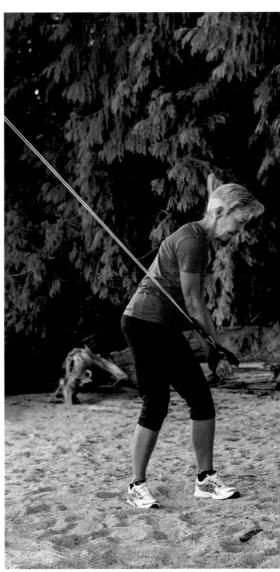

LOW-HIGH CHOP

Much like the high-low chop, this exercise targets your transverse abdominis and oblique muscles. It's usually a bit more challenging than the high-low chop, so you may need to use slightly less resistance.

Stand with your feet hip width apart, to the left of a resistance band anchored just below knee height. Hold both resistance handles together. Start with your arms straight and extended to your right, knees slightly bent.

Using your core muscles to initiate the movement (your arms should feel like they're just going along for the ride), move the band handles in a smooth arc to your left, ending with your hands at about head height.

Perform all reps on one side, then switch sides.

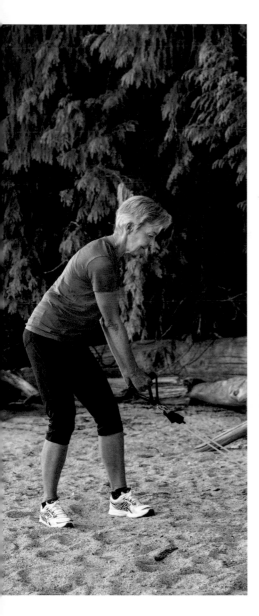
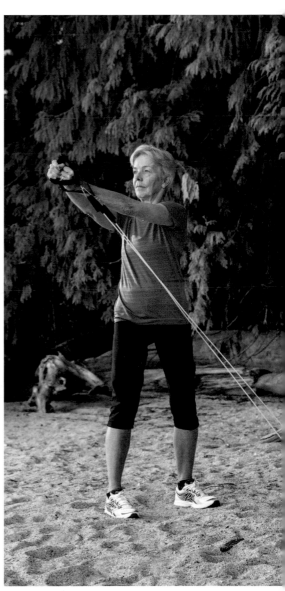

MOUNTAIN CLIMBER

This version of the mountain climber is slower and more core-focused than its common bodyweight-only counterpart, which is usually performed as a cardio conditioning exercise. Adding a mini-band builds strength in your hips, and helps you focus on using good form throughout the movement.

Start in a push-up position, with your hands and toes touching the ground, and a mini-band looped around your feet. Your hands should be directly under your shoulders, and your torso and legs should form a straight line. Make sure your head is in line with your spine; you should be looking at the ground, not directly ahead of you.

Brace your abs and bring your right knee to your chest. Keep the toes of your right foot off the ground. Hold the contracted position briefly, then return to the start position and repeat on the other side. Alternate sides with each rep.

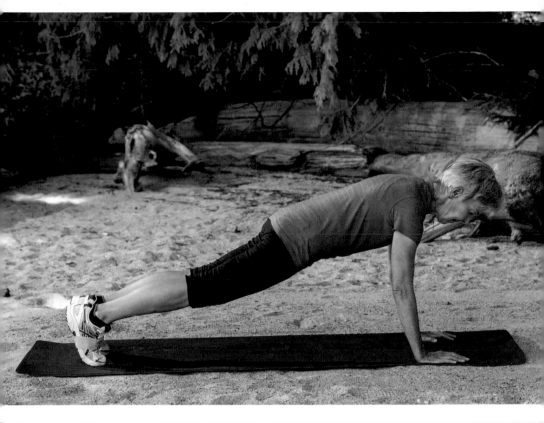

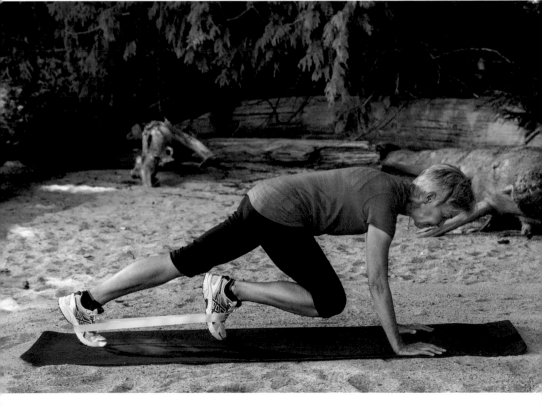

PALLOF PRESS

The Pallof press is an anti-rotational movement that will help you build a stable core. One of the main functions of your core is to resist rotation and maintain rigidity through the trunk and hips while your arms and legs engage in movement. This translates into power in sport performance, including weight lifting or powerlifting, boxing, golfing, and more.

Stand to the right of your anchor point, set to about waist height, with your feet shoulder-width apart and knees slightly bent. Hold both resistance band handles in your left hand, and place your right hand on top of your left. Start with your hands a few inches in front of your chest, with tension on the resistance band.

Press the resistance band handles straight ahead, keeping your arms at chest height. Don't let your arms shift to the left during this movement, and keep your hips square (you'll feel them want to rotate, due to the band tension coming from one side).

To make the Pallof press more challenging, bring your feet closer together. A narrower stance forces your core to work harder to keep your torso in the correct position and to prevent your hips from rotating. Perform all reps on one side, then switch sides.

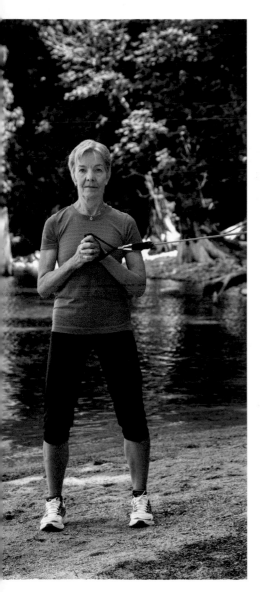
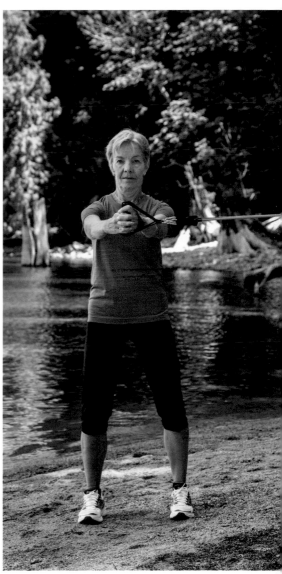

PSOAS MARCH

This deceptively simple exercise for the psoas (one of the hip flexor muscles) helps improve lumbo-pelvic stability. The hip flexors are often tight, especially for those of us who spend a lot of time sitting. Often it's muscle weakness that makes them tense, so make sure to incorporate this exercise into your regular routine. It can also help prevent and decrease low back pain, and increase core strength.

Lie on your back with a mini-band around your feet. Bend your legs so your thighs are perpendicular to the ground, and your knees are bent at 90 degrees. Flex your feet so your toes point upward. Press your low back into the ground, using your abdominal muscles to maintain that position throughout the exercise.

Slowly straighten your right leg toward the ground, pressing your right foot into the band, and keeping your left leg bent. You should feel the hip flexor muscles in your left hip working. Pause when your right leg is fully extended, then slowly return to the start position. Then straighten your left leg as your right hip flexor resists the band's tension. Alternate sides with each rep.

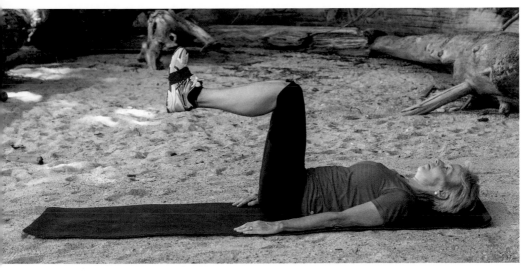

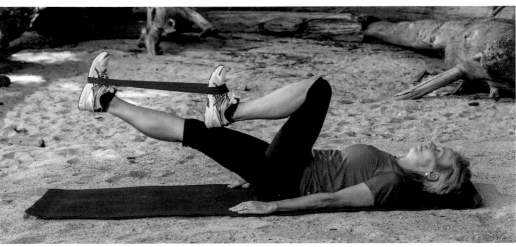

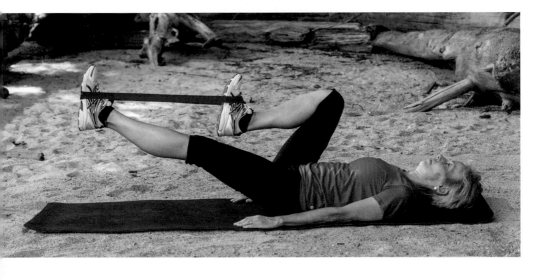

SIDE PLANK ROW

This challenging side plank variation will work your obliques, gluteus medius (the side of your glutes), shoulders, and back. Start by practicing this move from your knees, as you see here. If you'd like a greater challenge, try it from your feet.

Set up a resistance band in an anchor point at about knee height. Facing the anchor point, get into a kneeling side plank position by propping yourself up on your left forearm (making sure your elbow is directly under your shoulder), stacking your right leg onto your left leg, bending both legs, and lifting your hips off the ground. Your body should form a straight line from your head to your knees.

You may need to perform a slight posterior pelvic tilt to maintain proper alignment. Do this by squeezing your glutes, bracing your abs, and flattening out the curve in your low back.

Hold both resistance band handles in your right hand, reaching your right arm out in front of you so it's completely straight. Make sure you feel tension on the band at this point. If not, adjust your position so you're slightly further away from the anchor point.

Maintaining the side plank position throughout your set, row the resistance band handles to the right side of your chest. Pause briefly, then return to the start position. Perform all reps on one side, then switch sides.

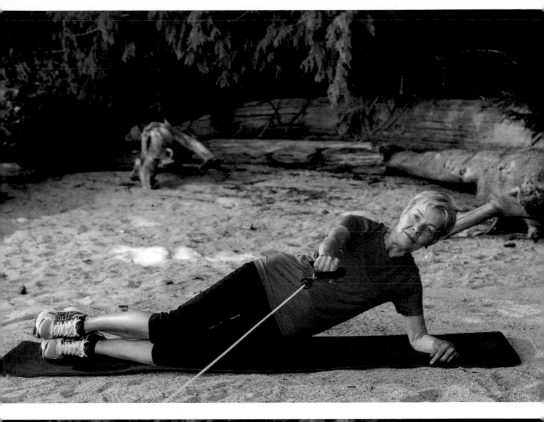
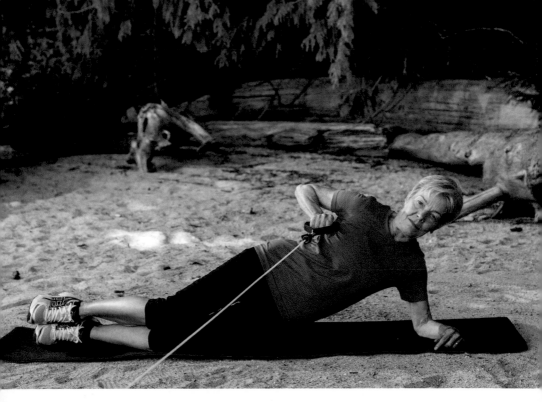

How to Create Your Own Resistance Band Workout Program

Now that you have an understanding of 50 different resistance band exercises, you'll learn how to put together a well-rounded workout program. Having a list of exercises is well and good, but it won't be of any use if you don't put it into action!

I'll first go over the six basic movement patterns that should be included in every training plan. I'll then show you how to create your own workout program, putting together resistance band exercises for between two and six workouts per week, depending upon your preference, goals, and available time.

THE SIX FUNDAMENTAL STRENGTH MOVEMENT PATTERNS

Squat

Research shows that squats are particularly effective at improving bone strength.[1] Squatting is an important and fundamental movement that improves strength and hip mobility, and has excellent carryover into daily movement patterns as well, like standing up from a seated position, or lifting objects from the ground. Squats can help increase your athletic performance in any sport that requires lower body power and strength (that is, most sports!).

---

1   M. P. Mosti et al. (2013). "Maximal strength training in postmenopausal women with osteoporosis or osteopenia," *Journal of Strength and Conditioning Research,* *27*(10), (2013): 2879–86. https://www.ncbi.nlm.nih.gov/pubmed/23287836, accessed December 30, 2017.

Squats you can perform with resistance bands include the banded squat on page 82.

Hip Hinge

Hip hinge movements train the muscles of the back of the body, often called the posterior chain. This includes the hamstrings, glutes, and low back. When you perform hip hinges, you should feel your hamstrings and glutes performing most of the work, as opposed to your quads or low back. Hip hinge strength exercises have many benefits, including improved posture, preventing and decreasing low back pain, and being able to lift objects off the ground with good form (i.e., without injuring your back!). The hip hinge is also the foundation of the athletic stance, in which you stand with your feet hip width apart, shoulders back, knees bent, and hips hinged behind you. The athletic stance prepares athletes for movement in any direction, and reduces the chance of injury.

The most well-known example of a hip hinge is the barbell deadlift. Kettlebell swings are another common example. You'll find a unique superband hip hinge on page 88. Other hip hinge examples are pull-throughs (page 96) and kickstand deadlifts (page 90).

Lunge

Lunges develop ankle, knee, and hip stability (which all translate into better balance), in addition to strengthening all the muscle groups of your legs.

You can perform lunges with countless different pieces of equipment, including using just your bodyweight. You can also add a loaded barbell on your back, or hold dumbbells or kettlebells.

When my chronic low back pain flares up and I want to train my lower body without loading my spine with exercises like barbell squats or deadlifts, I'll do bodyweight lunges for high reps: performing walking lunges around a 400-meter track. That's about 450 lunges!

You'll find an example of a resistance band lunge on page 106 (described as a variation of the split squat).

Upper Body Push

Upper body push movements focus on the pectoral, deltoid, and triceps muscles. Horizontal push movements primarily use the pectoral muscles, like incline push-ups (page 54) or the resistance band chest press (page 42). In the gym, horizontal push movements include the barbell or dumbbell bench press. Vertical push movements focus on the deltoids, like the overhead press (page 64) and the Arnold press (page 32), which can both be performed with dumbbells as well.

Upper Body Pull

These movements work mainly the upper back muscles (including the rhomboids and latissimus dorsi), but also work the biceps and forearm muscles. Upper body pull movements are crucial to maintaining good posture, healthy shoulders, and a pain-free back and neck.

Horizontal pulls include the standing row (page 70) and standing wide row (page 72). In the gym, this would include the seated cable row. Vertical pulls involve starting with your arms overhead, as in pull-ups and chin-ups. The kneeling pull-down (page 56) is an example of a resistance band vertical pull.

Plank

In weight lifting, the sixth fundamental movement pattern is weighted carries (also called loaded carries). This involves picking up heavy objects such as kettlebells or dumbbells, and slowly walking with them for a set distance, keeping all the upper body and core muscles engaged. The goal is to carry the equivalent of your total bodyweight, so this is quite challenging!

In resistance band training, we don't have the option of carrying very heavy objects, so I've updated the sixth fundamental movement to be a plank. Planks are a very important core-strengthening exercise. When performed correctly, they can help us decrease low back pain and prevent injury. For examples, see the side plank row on page 128 and the mountain climber on page 122.

How to Design Your Resistance Band Training Program

WARMING UP BEFORE YOUR WORKOUTS

To prevent injury or muscle strains, make sure you warm up before each strength training workout. I recommend five minutes of moderate intensity cardio activity, like jogging, power walking, cycling on a stationary bike, or rowing. For the first two or three exercises of your strength workout, perform a warm-up set. For example, if the first two moves of your workout are a resistance band chest press and banded squats, perform 10 to 12 reps of the chest press with a resistance level a few steps lighter than what you'd normally use, and perform 10 to 12 squats with no added mini-band.

You can also include a few resistance band moves in your warm-up. Here are four suggestions that get your muscles ready for your workout:

Band pull-apart (page 34)
Hip hinge (page 88)
Clamshell (page 84)
Lateral walk (page 92)

CARDIO FIRST OR STRENGTH TRAINING FIRST?

If steady-state cardio activity, like running, swimming, cycling, rowing, etc., is part of your workout plan, make sure you perform cardio *after* strength training, or separate from it. If you're strength training and completing cardio activity in the same workout, do your strength training first (after a short warm-up), and cardio afterward. Strength training takes more focus and attention to exercise form than cardio, so you want to be mentally "fresh" for your strength moves.

To get the most out of your strength training workouts, you need to be able to challenge yourself at about a 7 out of 10 on the perceived exertion scale (where 1 is sitting on the couch, and 10 is all-out effort). If you do cardio first, you'd deplete your energy and muscular endurance, and possibly not be able to use as much resistance during strength training.

Another option is to separate cardio from strength training. You can perform these activities on separate days, or do one activity in the morning, and the other in the evening.

REPS AND SETS

A rep is one performance of a single exercise. For example, one rep of a squat means performing one squat. Ten reps is ten squats. A set is the number of repetitions performed without stopping. For example, "3 sets of 10 reps" for squats means performing 10 squats, taking a short break (or performing another exercise), completing another set of 10 squats, taking another short break, and performing a third round of 10 squats.

Some research shows that higher weights with lower reps and higher reps with lower weights are equally effective at building muscle, especially in beginner strength trainees.[1] Much of this research uses very high rep

---

1   C. G. Mitchell et al. "Resistance exercise load does not determine training-mediated hypertrophic gains in young men." *Journal of Applied Physiology, 113*(1) (2012): 71–77. https://www.ncbi.nlm.nih.gov/pubmed/22518835.

ranges, like sets of 20 to 30 reps. This can be highly uncomfortable to perform, and it takes much longer to complete a workout with reps this high, compared to a rep range of, say, 10 to 15. Assuming you're challenging yourself appropriately, the rep range of 10 to 15 is essentially a "sweet spot." It's not too low, where you'd need a very heavy weight (and beginners would be putting themselves at risk for injury), and not too high, where it would take half the day just to do your strength workout.

Rep schemes will differ based on individual goals. Endurance athletes must be able to perform athletically for long stretches of time, and thus may strength train at higher rep ranges. Powerlifters, on the other hand, compete in events that require a great amount of strength in performing single reps with heavy weights. They will vary their rep ranges within their training programs, but generally don't perform a lot of high-rep work, other than for accessory movements or activation exercises.

For strength training with resistance bands, we usually aim for 3 to 4 sets of between 10 and 15 reps. Resistance bands lend themselves well to medium- and high-rep work, rather than low-rep (and heavy weight) work.

STRAIGHT SETS, SUPERSETS, TRI-SETS, AND CIRCUITS

There are many different ways of performing strength training sets. A straight set is performing sets of an exercise without alternating it with another exercise, taking a short rest break in between sets.

For example, 3 sets of 10 squats performed as straight sets would look like this:

Set 1: 10 squats
[short rest]

Set 2: 10 squats
[short rest]

Set 3: 10 squats

Straight sets are often used in specific training programs like powerlifting, where a trainee may be working on one lift at a time (bench press, deadlift, or squat). Straight sets can also be convenient for moves that require more setup, or when training in a shared space that makes alternating between two or three exercises difficult.

Supersets are two exercises performed in an alternating manner: one set of Exercise A, then a set of Exercise B, then back to Exercise A. If a short rest is required, it's usually taken after both exercises have been completed.

When creating your own workout programs, keep in mind it's easier to superset exercises that won't require you to move your resistance band anchor point higher or lower after each exercise. For example, pairing a low-high chop, which requires a low anchor point, with a kneeling pull-down, which requires a high anchor point, will waste a lot of time! Try pairing exercises that use the same anchor point (like a chest press and a standing row, for example), or use exercise pairs where only one move requires an anchor point (for example, pair a split squat, where the resistance band is anchored under your foot, with a torso rotation, which requires an anchor point; or pair a mini-band exercise with a resistance band exercise that uses an anchor).

For example, 3 sets of 10 reps for squats and chest press, performed as a superset, would look like this:

Set 1:
10 squats
10 chest presses
[short rest, if required]

Set 2:
10 squats
10 chest presses
[short rest, if required]

Set 3:
10 squats
10 chest presses

Supersets can be used to train different muscle groups (e.g., a lunge that works the lower body paired with a chest press that works the upper body), or the same muscle group (e.g., an overhead press paired with a lateral raise; both work the deltoids). When supersets are used to train different muscle groups, they can save a lot of time and shorten your workout. Rather than taking a break between sets of lunges, for example, you'd be performing chest presses. Your legs are getting a break, but you're still continuing with your workout. Performing supersets in this manner also helps keep your heart rate elevated throughout your workout.

Supersets are one of the most common methods of performing strength workouts. It's efficient, effective, and doesn't require a lot of setup as you're performing only two exercises at a time. The vast majority of the programs I create for my clients involve supersets.

Similar to supersets, a tri-set rotates between three exercises instead of two. The goal is to complete all three exercises before resting. Much like supersets, when you're designing your own programs, it's easiest to choose exercises that won't involve moving your resistance band anchor point during each tri-set.

For example, 3 sets of 10 reps for squats, chest press, and standing rows, performed as a tri-set, would look like this:

Set 1:
10 squats
10 chest presses
10 standing rows
[short rest, if required]

Set 2:
10 squats
10 chest presses
10 standing rows
[short rest, if required]

Set 3:
10 squats
10 chest presses
10 standing rows

Circuits involve performing more than three exercises in a row. Typically used with cardiovascular exercises or conditioning exercises (a combination of strength and cardio), circuits can be based on reps, but they're often timed. For example, you might perform five exercises for 45 seconds each, with a 15-second rest between each exercise.

Here's an example of one set of a 5-minute circuit:

Squats for 45 seconds
[15-second rest]

Chest press for 45 seconds
[15-second rest]

Standing row for 45 seconds
[15-second rest]

Reverse lunges for 45 seconds
[15-second rest]

Overhead press for 45 seconds
[15-second rest]

After completing one set, you'd start back at the top with squats, and work your way back down to overhead press. Three sets of this particular circuit would take fifteen minutes.

I suggest creating strength training programs for yourself that are based mostly on supersets, but do throw in tri-sets and circuits on a regular basis to make sure you're challenging your strength and endurance in different ways.

COMPOUND VERSUS ISOLATION MOVEMENTS

Compound movements involve more than one joint, while isolation movements use only one joint. Push-ups, squats, lunges, deadlifts, and overhead presses are compound exercises, while biceps curls, lateral raises, hip extensions, and triceps kickbacks are isolation movements.

Compound movements should be prioritized in your programming. If there's time left over at the end of your program, and you've trained with compound movements all the major muscle groups being worked on a certain day, isolation movements can be helpful in building muscle, evening out strength imbalances between your left and right sides, and getting that sought-after "pumped" muscle feeling (which is increased blood flow to your muscles).

Make sure you perform compound movements first in your workouts, rather than tiring out certain muscles with isolation movements, and then attempting to recruit them again for a compound lift. For example, perform chest presses (which involve pecs, triceps, and deltoids) before performing triceps kickbacks. Perform standing rows (which involve the muscles of the back and biceps) before performing biceps curls. And perform squats (which involve the quads, glutes, and hamstrings) before performing hip extensions (which work just the glutes).

TRAINING SPLITS

A "training split" describes how working different muscle groups is distributed across your workouts each week. A full body training split means working all your major muscle groups each time you work out. An upper-lower training split means alternating between working your upper body on one day, and your lower body the next.

Bodybuilders will often use a body part split, for example working chest on Monday, back on Tuesday, shoulders on Wednesday, legs on Thursday, and biceps and triceps on Friday. Note that this is not an effective training split for most people, since you're training each muscle group only once a week.

There is no "one size fits all" approach to training splits—or anything else in fitness, for that matter! Your ideal training split will be based on your goals, schedule, and individual variables like recovery time, any injuries or conditions you're working around, and body type.

The two training splits I most often recommend are full-body and upper-lower. If you're working out two to three days per week, create a program that includes all your major muscle groups in each workout. If you're working out four to five days a week, you may want to try an upper-lower split.

The upper-lower split is generally seen as more advanced than the full-body split, since the total training volume (the amount of reps, sets, and weight) for each muscle group is higher. For example, in a full-body workout program, you're training chest, back, shoulders, quads, hamstrings, glutes, and abs on the same day. If your workout involves three sets of eight different exercises, you'll do one or two exercises for each muscle group (there's some overlap; for example, a deadlift works the hamstrings and also the glutes, and a lunge works the quads but also the glutes).

In an upper-lower split, since you're training only upper body or only lower body at one time, if your workout contains three sets of eight different exercises, you're now doing eight exercises all for your upper body, or eight exercises all for your lower body. That's a lot more volume than training all your muscle groups in the same session, and generally makes for a more challenging workout.

In this type of training split, there's more room for isolation movements compared to a full-body training split. In two- or three-day training splits, you'd need to train all your major muscle groups in each workout. If you need to train each major muscle group in a single workout, you won't be left with much room for single-joint isolation moves like biceps curls and triceps extensions. When I create strength training programs for my clients, isolation moves typically appear only in training splits of four or more days per week.

If you're just starting out with strength training, try a full-body routine for the first month or two, while you get familiar with the movements and build up a good baseline of strength. Then, if you have four days per week available to train, you can try the upper-lower split.

CORE TRAINING

Our abdominal and low back muscles (collectively the "core") can be trained more frequently than other muscle groups. You'll notice that in all the workout programs I've created on the following pages, I've included at least one core exercise—even in the six-days-per-week workout program.

In this context, you're performing one or two core strength exercises per day, rather than a dedicated core workout with a higher volume of exercises and reps. If you prefer performing core-only workouts, try creating a ten- or fifteen-minute core routine that you perform three or four times per week. At the end of the sample workouts section, you'll see three suggested core workouts.

In general, I try to place core moves near the end of strength workout programs. During the first part of a strength workout, you'll be performing compound movements (like squats, single leg deadlifts, push-ups, overhead presses, etc.) that require core activation to maintain proper form. This is especially the case when you perform strength movements with other types of non-resistance band equipment, like squatting with a loaded barbell on your back, performing kettlebell swings, or bench pressing with heavy dumbbells. If you tire out your core muscles before engaging in any of your compound lifts, you run the risk of losing good form, which may lead to injury.

Sample Workout Programs

TWO WORKOUTS PER WEEK

Training all of our major muscle groups twice a week is the minimum recommended by the US Office of Disease Prevention and Health Promotion and the Canadian Society for Exercise Physiology. If you have only two days available each week for strength training, you can certainly see benefits.

Day 1

Perform exercises as supersets. Aim for 3 sets of 12 to 15 reps (each side, where applicable), making sure rep number 10 feels very challenging.
Workout time: approximately 40 minutes (with minimal breaks).

1. Chest press	Page 42
2. Standing row	Page 70
3. Glute bridge	Page 86
4. Lateral walk	Page 92
5. Arnold press	Page 32
6. Banded squat	Page 82
7. Mountain climber	Page 122
8. Side plank row	Page 128

Day 2

Perform exercises as supersets. Aim for 3 sets of 10 to 12 reps (each side, where applicable), making sure rep number 7 feels very challenging.

Workout time: approximately 40 minutes (with minimal breaks).

1. Kneeling pull-down   Page 56
2. Split squat   Page 106

3. Chest press   Page 42
4. Kickstand deadlift   Page 90

5. Overhead press   Page 64
6. Superband hip hinge   Page 88

7. Bicycle crunch   Page 116
8. High-low chop   Page 118

THREE WORKOUTS PER WEEK

With three workouts per week, make sure you're training all your major muscle groups during each workout. You'll see more strength and muscle gain benefits than training only twice a week. This training split is very useful for people who use strength training to improve their performance and prevent injury in other sports. My triathlete, competitive cyclist, or long-distance runner clients, for example, typically strength train three days per week to leave room in their schedules for their other training. Three-day-a-week training splits are most common during their race seasons; many of these athletes will transition to a four-day-a-week strength training routine in their off-seasons.

Day 1

Perform exercises as supersets. Aim for 3 sets of 10 to 12 reps (each side, where applicable), making sure rep number 7 feels very challenging.

Workout time: approximately 40 minutes (with minimal breaks).

1.	Quadruped kickback	Page 98
2.	Kickstand deadlift	Page 90
3.	Face pull	Page 44
4.	Incline push-up	Page 54
5.	Standing row	Page 70
6.	Banded squat	Page 82
7.	Mountain climber	Page 122
8.	Bicycle crunch	Page 116

Day 2

Perform exercises as tri-sets. Aim for 3 sets of 10 to 12 reps (each side, where applicable), making sure rep number 7 feels very challenging.

Workout time: approximately 40 minutes (with minimal breaks).

1.	Superband side lunge	Page 112
2.	Pull-through	Page 96
3.	Superband hip hinge	Page 88
4.	Incline chest press	Page 52
5.	Arnold press	Page 32
6.	Standing wide row	Page 72
7.	Torso rotation	Page 114
8.	Psoas march	Page 126
9.	Mountain climber	Page 122

Day 3

Perform exercises as a circuit. You'll cycle through all the exercises from number one to number nine, then start back at number one. You won't need a resistance band anchor point for this workout, so you can quickly switch between different resistance bands.

Use an interval timer: 45 seconds of work, followed by 15 seconds of rest. Complete 4 rounds of the circuit.

Workout time: 36 minutes.

1. Incline push-up   Page 54
2. Glute bridge   Page 86
3. Bicycle crunch   Page 116
4. Banded squat   Page 82
5. Lateral walk   Page 92
6. Band pull-apart   Page 34
7. Overhead press   Page 64
8. Biceps curl   Page 40
9. Bent-over rear delt fly   Page 36

FOUR WORKOUTS PER WEEK

Splitting your workouts across four days per week gives you more options for training splits. You could train all your major muscle groups each time, especially if you're more advanced and your muscles have a shorter recovery time. What I'd suggest, however, is splitting your workouts into upper body and lower body, performing two of each during each week. Core exercises can be included in each workout.

For example, you could train upper body on Monday, lower body on Tuesday, take a rest day Wednesday, then train upper body on Thursday and lower body on Friday.

Day 1: Upper Body

Perform exercises as supersets. Aim for 3 sets of 10 to 12 reps (each side, where applicable), making sure rep number 7 feels very challenging.

Workout time: approximately 40 minutes (with minimal breaks).

1. Superband seated row   Page 76
2. Incline push-up   Page 54

3. Arnold press   Page 32
4. Face pull   Page 44

5. High curl   Page 50
6. Overhead extension   Page 62

7. High-low chop   Page 118
8. Mountain climber   Page 122

Day 2: Lower Body

Perform exercises as supersets. Aim for 3 sets of 10 to 12 reps (each side, where applicable), making sure rep number 7 feels very challenging. For lower body workouts, I usually include slightly fewer exercises than upper body workouts, because so many lower body movements are unilateral (single-sided) and reps need to be completed on each side separately.

Workout time: approximately 40 minutes (with minimal breaks).

1. Superband deadlift   Page 108
2. Split squat   Page 106

3. Banded squat   Page 82
4. Mountain climber   Page 122

5. Clamshell   Page 84
6. Lateral walk   Page 92

Day 3: Upper Body

Perform exercises as supersets. Aim for 3 sets of 12 to 15 reps (each side, where applicable), making sure rep number 10 feels very challenging.

Workout time: approximately 40 minutes (with minimal breaks).

1. Standing wide row   Page 72
2. Overhead press   Page 64

3. Chest press   Page 42
4. Band pull-apart   Page 34

5. Biceps curl   Page 40
6. Triceps kickback   Page 78

7. Lateral raise   Page 58
8. Side plank row   Page 128

Day 4: Lower Body

Perform exercises as supersets. Aim for 3 sets of 12 to 15 reps (each side, where applicable), making sure rep number 10 feels very challenging.

Workout time: approximately 40 minutes (with minimal breaks).

1. Lying abduction   Page 94
2. Glute bridge   Page 86

3. Banded squat   Page 82
4. Superband single leg press Page 110

5. Pull-through   Page 96
6. Low-high chop   Page 120

FIVE TO SIX WORKOUTS PER WEEK

Many of our beginner and intermediate clients prefer shorter daily workouts, rather than longer workouts a few times per week. For example, you could complete a 15-minute full-body routine five days a week, rather than performing three 25-minute workouts. The total minutes each week in both cases is 75. For those working to establish a daily habit of intentional exercise, shorter and more frequent workouts can be useful.

More advanced strength trainees will often complete five or more full (40- to 60-minute) workouts each week. My own training includes five 45- to 60-minute strength sessions per week: two upper body workouts, two lower body workouts, and one full-body workout per week (plus two to three cardio sessions).

Those completing shorter workouts each day may wish to perform full-body workouts each time. In most cases, however, I'd split your weekly workouts into upper, lower, and full-body routines, with core exercises included in at least three workouts per week.

Beginner Five- or Six-Day Workout Program
Day 1: Lower Body
Perform exercises as supersets. Aim for 3 sets of 10 to 12 reps (each side, where applicable), making sure rep number 7 feels very challenging.
Workout time: 15–20 minutes (with minimal breaks).

1.	Single leg hip extension	Page 104
2.	Single leg glute bridge	Page 102
3.	Superband side lunge	Page 112
4.	Lying abduction	Page 94

Day 2: Upper Body

Perform exercises as supersets. Aim for 3 sets of 12 to 15 reps (each side, where applicable), making sure rep number 10 feels very challenging.

Workout time: 15–20 minutes (with minimal breaks).

1. Bent-over row   Page 38
2. Incline chest press   Page 52

3. Overhead press   Page 64
4. Bicycle crunch   Page 116

Day 3: Lower Body

Perform exercises as supersets. Aim for 3 sets of 12 to 15 reps (each side, where applicable), making sure rep number 7 feels very challenging.

Workout time: 15–20 minutes (with minimal breaks).

1. Kickstand deadlift   Page 90
2. Split squat   Page 106

3. Low-high chop   Page 120
4. Psoas march   Page 126

Day 4: Upper Body

Perform exercises as supersets. Aim for 3 sets of 10 to 12 reps (each side, where applicable), making sure rep number 7 feels very challenging.

Workout time: 15–20 minutes (with minimal breaks).

1. Kneeling pull-down   Page 56
2. Incline push-up   Page 54

3. Arnold press   Page 32
4. Side plank row   Page 128

Day 5: Full Body

Perform exercises as a circuit. You'll cycle through all the exercises from number one to number five, then start back at number one. You won't need a resistance band anchor point for this workout, so you can quickly switch between different resistance bands.

Use an interval timer: 45 seconds of work, followed by 15 seconds of rest. Complete 4 rounds of the circuit.

Workout time: 20 minutes.

1. Bent-over rear delt fly   Page 36
2. Banded squat   Page 82
3. Mountain climber   Page 122
4. Overhead press   Page 64
5. Bicycle crunch   Page 116

Optional Day 6: Full Body

Perform exercises as supersets. Aim for 3 sets of 12 to 15 reps (each side, where applicable), making sure rep number 7 feels very challenging.

Workout time: 15–20 minutes (with minimal breaks).

1. Chest press   Page 42
2. Split squat   Page 106

3. Face pull   Page 44
4. High-low chop   Page 118

Advanced Five or Six-Day Workout Program

Day 1: Lower Body

Perform exercises as supersets. Aim for 3 sets of 10 to 12 reps (each side, where applicable), making sure rep number 7 feels very challenging. **Workout time:** 40–50 minutes (with minimal breaks).

1. Single leg hip extension Page 104
2. Pull-through   Page 96

3. Superband hip hinge   Page 88
4. Quadruped kickback   Page 98

5. Glute bridge   Page 86
6. Lateral walk   Page 92

7. Banded squat   Page 82
8. Torso rotation   Page 114

Day 2: Upper Body

Perform exercises as supersets. Aim for 3 sets of 12 to 15 reps (each side, where applicable), making sure rep number 10 feels very challenging. **Workout time:** 40–50 minutes (with minimal breaks).

1. Bent-over row   Page 38
2. Chest press   Page 42

3. Overhead press   Page 64
4. Straight arm pulldown   Page 74

5. Triceps press-down   Page 80
6. High curl   Page 50

7. Mountain climber	Page 122
8. High-low chop	Page 118

Day 3: Lower Body

Perform exercises as supersets. Aim for 3 sets of 12 to 15 reps (each side, where applicable), making sure rep number 7 feels very challenging.
Workout time: 40–50 minutes (with minimal breaks).

1. Kickstand deadlift	Page 90
2. Split squat	Page 106
3. Superband single leg press	Page 110
4. Clamshell	Page 84
5. Lateral walk	Page 92
6. Glute bridge	Page 86
7. Psoas march	Page 126
8. Bicycle crunch	Page 116

Day 4: Upper Body

Perform exercises as supersets. Aim for 3 sets of 10 to 12 reps (each side, where applicable), making sure rep number 7 feels very challenging.
Workout time: 40–50 minutes (with minimal breaks).

1. Kneeling pull-down	Page 56
2. Incline push-up	Page 54
3. Arnold press	Page 32
4. Standing row	Page 70
5. Low curl	Page 60
6. Overhead extension	Page 62

7. Pec fly   Page 66
8. Pallof press   Page 124

Day 5: Full Body

Perform exercises as a circuit. You'll cycle through all the exercises from number one to number nine, then start back at number one. You won't need a resistance band anchor point for this workout, so you can quickly switch between different resistance bands.

Use an interval timer: 45 seconds of work, followed by 15 seconds of rest. Complete 4 rounds of the circuit.

Workout time: 36 minutes.

1. Bent-over rear delt fly   Page 36
2. Incline push-up   Page 54
3. Banded squat   Page 82
4. Glute bridge   Page 86
5. Mountain climber   Page 122
6. Overhead press   Page 64
7. Biceps curl   Page 40
8. Bent-over row   Page 38
9. Psoas march   Page 126

Optional Day 6: Full Body

Perform exercises as supersets. Aim for 3 sets of 12 to 15 reps (each side, where applicable), making sure rep number 7 feels very challenging. Workout time: 40–50 minutes (with minimal breaks).

1. Chest press   Page 42
2. Split squat   Page 106

3. Pallof press   Page 124
4. Superband side lunge   Page 112

CORE WORKOUT EXAMPLES

If you prefer performing core-only workouts instead of incorporating core movements into your other strength programs, here are three workouts to try. They take between nine and fifteen minutes, so they can be added to the end of your regular strength workouts, or they can be performed on their own. Completing a core-only workout is more challenging than many people think, especially when you're using an interval timer and your rest breaks are limited!

Core workout 1

Complete this workout as a tri-set, cycling through all the exercises from number one to number three, then start back at number one. Perform each exercise for 45 seconds, followed by 15 seconds of rest. It's most convenient to use an interval timer app, so you can "set it and forget it," rather than having to reset a timer throughout your workout. If at first you're unable to complete reps nonstop for each 45-second set, just perform as many reps as you can, taking breaks when necessary.

Workout time: 9 minutes.

Core workout 2

Perform exercises as supersets. Aim for 3 sets of 12 to 15 reps (each side, where applicable), making sure rep number 7 feels very challenging.
Workout time: 10–15 minutes.

1. Low-high chop   Page 120
2. Side plank row   Page 128

3. Torso rotation   Page 114
4. Bicycle crunch   Page 116

Core workout 3

Perform exercises as supersets. Aim for 3 sets of 12 to 15 reps (each side, where applicable), making sure rep number 7 feels very challenging.
Workout time: 10–15 minutes.

1. High-low chop   Page 118
2. Mountain climber   Page 122

3. Pallof press   Page 124
4. Psoas march   Page 126

How to Ensure Your Muscles Recover Effectively from Strength Training

As beneficial as strength training is, keep in mind that it's not the whole story when it comes to gaining strength, changing your body composition, and improving your athletic ability and day-to-day function. If you're not supporting your strength training routine with other basic elements of muscle recovery, you may be hindering your results. Make sure you're eating a nutrient-dense diet, getting adequate sleep each night, and staying hydrated to ensure you're fully recovering your muscles from your workouts.

Muscle recovery is just as important as physical activity; they go hand-in-hand when it comes to taking care of your body and achieving your fitness goals. By focusing on both exercise and recovery, you'll be getting the most out of your active lifestyle.

When you work out at a challenging intensity, you're creating microscopic tears in your muscle fibers. Don't worry, that's a good thing! This means your muscles need time between workouts to repair themselves. It's this between-workout time during which your muscles rebuild and gain density and strength. Your workout may last only 45 minutes, but it's what you do in the next 48 hours that can support or hinder getting the results you want. The general rule for strength training is to leave 48 hours between training the same muscle group. You could, for example, complete a full body circuit on Mondays, Wednesdays, and Fridays. Or you could train upper body on Mondays, lower body on Tuesdays, upper body on Thursdays, and lower body on Fridays.

As you become more experienced with strength training, your muscles won't need as much recovery time. Elite athletes often train the same muscle groups daily, as their recovery windows are much smaller. Even non-athletes who have been strength training consistently for many years will have shorter recovery times than novices.

With cardio activities such as running or swimming, there's less of a consensus among fitness professionals as to how long muscles take to recover. If you're training regularly, keep tabs on how your body feels and whether it's telling you it needs rest. Take at least one day off from intense exercise each week, and try to mix up your activities so you're not always doing the same thing.

TAKE A REST DAY

A rest day means a day without intense exercise in order to give your body time to recover from regular training. Rest days are appropriate for you if you work out at a moderate-to-high intensity four to six times per week. Someone who works out once a week for ten minutes does not need designated rest days. But someone training on most days of the week at a high intensity most certainly needs at least one rest day per week.

ACTIVE RECOVERY

If you regularly train at a high intensity, active recovery days are often helpful. They're especially useful for those crazy fitness nuts who just can't deal with a day that involves no workout. In contrast to a rest day—where you're not doing any physical activity—active recovery means engaging in a low-intensity activity that differs from your regular workout activities.

For example, if you're a serious swimmer, your active recovery day might be going for an easy 20-minute bike ride. If you train with resistance bands regularly, your active recovery might be going for a walk. The idea is to do a very light, low-impact activity for a short period of time.

Active recovery is a good way to relax, and to increase blood circulation. Increased circulation is thought to improve muscle recovery.[1]

FOAM ROLLING

Self-myofascial release (the fancy term for using a foam roller) can be a great muscle recovery method. It can also help improve your mobility. Foam rolling is most often used as a form of self-massage, working out the soreness and tight spots in our muscles. It's much more economical than seeing a masseuse, athletic trainer, or other body-worker; plus, you're able to control precisely where to apply pressure, and how much.

A foam roller is a cylinder of dense foam, usually six inches in diameter, and typically one or three feet. You place the foam roller on the floor and use your own bodyweight to apply pressure to various muscle groups, slowly rolling back and forth across each muscle.

MASSAGE

Massage (via massage therapy or sports massage) is an excellent way to recover your muscles and leave them feeling much less sore and stiff. You'll also increase immune function[2], circulation, and joint mobility while you're at it. Massage is a great method of preventing problems in the first place, including muscle knots, tension headaches, and various forms of injury. Most serious athletes have regular massages as part of their muscle recovery plans. A qualified massage therapist will be better able to focus on precisely the muscles in your body that require work, compared to foam

1   D. P. Micklewright, R. Beneke, V. Gladwell, & M. H. Sellens. "Blood lactate removal using combined massage and active recovery," *Medicine & Science in Sports & Exercise, 35*(5), (2003): p. S317.
2   M. H. Rapaport, Schettler, P., & Bresee, C. "A preliminary study of the effects of a single session of Swedish massage on hypothalamic-pituitary-adrenal and immune function in normal individuals," *Journal of Alternative and Complementary Medicine, 16*(1), (2010): p. 1079–1088.

rolling on your own. Foam rolling is still very important—in part because it's so accessible—but ideally you'd use foam rolling to "fill in the gaps" between seeing a massage practitioner on a regular basis.

Even though foam rolling is often seen as a substitute for massage, foam rolling offers only compression of the body's tissues. Massage has the added benefit of also being able to separate layers of tissue from each other. For example, it's generally not recommended to foam roll the IT band (running along the outer thigh from the hip to the knee) or the low back. However, these areas can be safely manipulated through massage, using different techniques.

STRETCHING

Stretching directly after a workout can help your muscles relax and release tension. The clinical research jury is still out as to whether stretching can help prevent muscle soreness in the days following a workout, but many people who work out regularly claim that it does. Make sure that you stretch when your muscles are warm, such as right after completing your workout, or after taking a hot shower. Stretching cold muscles—like at the beginning of a workout—can increase your risk of tears, strains, and pulls. It's also been shown to decrease physical performance.

Make sure that your stretching sessions are pain free. Stretch slowly, relax your muscles, and only go so far as to feel a pulling, and perhaps a very slight burning sensation, in the muscle(s) you're stretching. If you stretch too far and cause pain, your muscles' defense mechanisms will kick in, in an effort to prevent injury. Muscles try to protect themselves by contracting, which is the opposite effect of the one you want from stretching.

Static stretching involves holding a stretch in the same position for a period of time, like sitting on the floor with your legs straight in front of you, reaching toward your toes to stretch the hamstrings. Dynamic stretching moves a particular muscle group through its entire range of motion in a fluid manner, which means you're moving during the stretch.

Examples of dynamic stretches are making circles with your arms (mobilizing the shoulder joint), or swinging one leg back and forth from the front of your body to the back while standing on the opposite foot (affecting the hip joint). Both static and dynamic stretches have benefits; work with a qualified fitness professional to ensure you're getting the most benefits from each. Stretching has many of the same benefits of yoga (not surprisingly, since they're both based on increasing flexibility), including increasing range of motion, preventing injury, and decreasing pain from muscle tightness.

YOGA

A few studies support the effectiveness of yoga in decreasing delayed onset muscle soreness (DOMS).[3] DOMS is the soreness you feel in the day or two after a workout (but keep in mind that DOMS is *not* a good indicator of workout effectiveness).

Yoga is also great for increasing flexibility and preventing injury. Many of us don't stretch for long enough (or at all!) after a workout to see any flexibility improvements over time. Yoga is a great way to get a healthy dose of flexibility and range of motion training. Also, many people find yoga more interesting than holding static stretches at the gym after a workout.

If you don't yet do yoga regularly, give it a try as a cross-training tool for your preferred physical activities.

SLEEP

Getting enough sleep is one of the most important things you can do to ensure your muscles recover and get stronger after a workout. During

---

3   C. A. Boyle et al. "The effects of yoga training and a single bout of yoga on delayed onset muscle soreness in the lower extremity," *Journal of Strength and Conditioning Research, 18*(4), (2004): p. 723–729.

deep sleep stages, your pituitary gland releases growth hormone that facilitates muscle repair and tissue growth. Growth hormone deficiency often leads to an increased risk for obesity, decreased muscle mass, and a lowered capacity for exercise.[4]

The exact relationship between exercise and sleep is still unclear, but a host of research studies have found a connection between sleep deprivation and decreased performance and recovery. Inadequate sleep is linked to having low energy levels and increased levels of the hormones that break down muscle[5], which is not something you want if you're looking to get—and keep—a lean body and a healthy metabolism!

Sleep is a prime time for the cells in our bodies to build new proteins (also known as protein synthesis).[6] Because protein is the building block of muscle, make sure you get your beauty sleep to keep your muscles healthy and functioning well.

Every person has his or her own sleep needs. There's no "gold standard" ideal amount of sleep to get each night, although most health authorities recommend between seven and nine hours per night. You may need to do some experimentation to find your optimal sleep length—you should be waking up well rested each morning.

Not sure how much sleep you need? You can find out, but you need about two weeks of a very flexible schedule. Perhaps you can take a sleep vacation! Go to bed at the same time every night, and don't set an alarm. Just wake up naturally. You might sleep for longer than normal the first few nights if you're chronically sleep deprived and need to catch up on sleep, but take note of what time you wake up during the second week. You'll likely wake up at a similar time each morning, at which point you've discovered the amount of sleep your body needs.

---

4   Reed, M. L., Merriam, G. R., and Kargi, A. Y. (2013). "Adult Growth Hormone Deficiency—Benefits, Side Effects, and Risks of Growth Hormone Replacement." Frontiers in Endocrinology, 4(64), https://www.ncbi.nlm.nih.gov/pmc/articles /PMC3671347

5   M. Datillo et al. "Sleep and muscle recovery: Endocrinological and molecular basis for a new and promising hypothesis," *Medical Hypotheses*, 77 (2), (2011): 220–222.

6   National Institutes of Health; National Institute of Neurological Disorders and Stroke "Brain basics: understanding sleep," 2007. http://www.ninds.nih.gov/disorders /brain_basics/understanding_sleep.htm#for_us

Strength Coaches on Using Resistance Bands with Their Clients

I asked four of my strength coach colleagues to share their views on the benefits of training with resistance bands, and how they use them with their clients.

Jennifer Fidder

Jennifer Fidder is an in-home and online personal trainer for women based out of Miami Beach, Florida. With a background in social psychology and educational science, she is able to provide a holistic approach to fitness that helps her clients become healthier, happier, and more confident.

"When I work in-person with clients, I love using resistance bands for their warm-ups. I will have them do arm swings with the bands, external rotations, shoulder extension, and/or band pull-aparts. These exercises help warm up the rotator cuffs and shoulder region in general. Strong rotator cuffs are essential to injury prevention, and adding some work to strengthen them during the warm-up provides a great set-up for other exercises during the session.

I also use bands to correct muscle imbalances or to address smaller muscles that could need some extra attention or activation like—in a lot of cases—the gluteus medius.

Resistance bands are great for travel! They are super lightweight and fit into any carry-on. You can also increase the efficacy of a dumbbell or barbell exercise by adding resistance bands. For example, you can add a loop resistance band above the knees when doing dumbbell or barbell squats.

Working with bands allows for a more fluid increase in resistance, compared to using dumbbells or barbells. This is especially beneficial for smaller or weaker muscles. For example, when performing front or lateral shoulder raises with dumbbells, an increase from 5 to 10 pounds can be very difficult. Some gyms will offer 7- or 8-pound dumbbells, but most smaller gyms or apartment gyms don't have that option. Using bands instead of dumbbells allows us to increase the resistance slowly, step by step.

One of my online clients is a busy human resources manager for a global company. She travels regularly—up to three weeks out of each month. While most of the hotels she stays at have gyms, she often simply doesn't have the time to go downstairs. She prefers to do her workout directly in her hotel room. She uses resistance bands she can hang in the door, or regular resistance bands without a door anchor. These are lightweight and fit easily in her suitcase or carry-on, which gives her a lot of workout flexibility. On long flights, she will also use loop bands while on the plane to keep her circulation up. Seated abductions or leg raises are just two of the exercises she can easily do while sitting in her seat."

Ren Jones

Ren Jones is a fitness professional certified in personal training, corrective exercise, nutrition, and online training. He's based in Charlotte, North Carolina, and specializes in coaching women.

"I love to use resistance bands for isometric resistance, especially when I have a client applying force in a different direction than the isometric resistance, as in the case of a half-kneeling Pallof press. This is such a great move for abs, obliques, erectors, and deep core stabilizers. That's one of my sneaky exercises to introduce to new clients who may still be lost in the mythology of the sit-up as the be-all, end-all of core training.

I love watching them go through a set of those for the first time! I typically use a resistance band with handles, looped around a fixed vertical object.

Another main way I use resistance bands with my clients is giving the awesome ladies I train a more "involved" assisted pull-up. The issue I have with the assisted pull-up machine is the fact that resting your knees (or feet) on a pad using a fixed plane of resistance that slides up and down a track completely removes the need for body control. Where's the fun in that, right?! But I can loop a resistance band (or two) over the top of a pull-up bar, and my client gets some great help with the lift while still having to learn posture in the movement and build her core to control the movement.

The most obvious advantage in regard to resistance bands is their portability. They're really convenient for travel. I guess you could try to travel with a set of dumbbells and maybe become an airport legend as you make your way onto the international airport watch list, but why not skip the cavity search?

Another big benefit, in my opinion, is the range of motion you can employ due to the fact that there's resistance, but no bulky weight. There's also an 'anchor,' but no fixed plane of motion. That allows some great, safe tension to be applied to some of the smaller muscles, like the rear (posterior) deltoids.

I have a client in her forties who was recovering from spinal stenosis due to an injury. Pallof press (page 124) was a great core exercise that helped build up the stabilizers around her spine, without having her engage in a bunch of goofy spinal flexion (like sit-ups). And even though she was very restricted in regard to overhead presses, as you might imagine with a low back injury, we were able to slowly introduce shoulder presses through utilizing bands. Now she's back to overhead pressing with dumbbells."

Dr. Emma Green

Dr. Green is an online coach and a freelance writer and editor. She helps people build healthy relationships with food, exercise, and their bodies.

"There are a few occasions when I use resistance bands with clients. The first is when they are not enjoying the gym anymore but want to continue to do resistance exercise. In this situation, I work with the client to find out their favorite and least favorite exercises, as well as the space and other tools they have available to create a program that suits them.

I also recommend resistance bands for clients who are travelling for an extended period. I discuss with them how much exercise is going to be both practical and enjoyable, and then design a program they can do while they're away. If they were enjoying the gym and/or are planning to rejoin a gym after travelling, I will ensure that the exercises more closely mirror those that would be done in the gym.

I think resistance bands can be beneficial psychologically because they don't involve numbers like dumbbells do. It can be easy to get caught up in the amount of weight and the number of sets and reps at the gym, which can detract from the enjoyment of the exercise. [Karina's note: many resistance band sets do come marked with weights like 10 pounds, 20 pounds, etc. However, those don't necessarily translate into actual weights, especially because you can alter the challenge level of a single band by moving closer or farther away from its anchor point.]

I also think they are useful to provide some variety within a routine. If people have been training for years with dumbbells and barbells, it can be refreshing to use some new tools. I find clients are surprised by how challenging resistance bands can be! One of my clients was recovering from a surgery and was not permitted to lift weights for a number of weeks afterwards, but was cleared by her doctor to do some more gentle movement. We worked together to build a program solely using resistance bands that mirrored her favorite exercises in the gym as much as possible. She ended up enjoying the program so much that she didn't ever rejoin the gym, and instead looked to other types of exercise to supplement her resistance band work, such as rowing and hiking. As personal trainers, it is easy to focus so much on the physiological aspects of exercise that we overlook the psychological elements. I think resistance bands are a great tool to have to help make programs more varied and enjoyable for clients."

Melody Schoenfeld

Melody is the owner of Flawless Fitness, a private training studio in Pasadena, California, and Evil Munky Enterprises, a custom steel fitness equipment manufacturer. She is the author of Pleasure Not Meating You *and is the 2019 NSCA Personal Trainer of the Year.*

"Resistance bands are extremely versatile. They're also cheap, convenient, and easy to travel with! While they make their way into most of my clients' training at some point, I find them particularly useful for clients with certain injuries or physical limitations (most recently, a client with a shattered wrist who had trouble gripping standard equipment). They can also come in handy for certain assistance exercises for powerlifting and strongman—either to add more weight to the top portion of a lift (e.g., a banded deadlift), or to remove weight from the bottom portion of a very heavy lift (e.g., a band-assisted bench press).

Many of my clients travel with bands because they can easily do resistance work in their hotel rooms. I often use high volume, light band work as a 'finisher' after my clients complete a workout."

Acknowledgments

I'd like to thank all the exceptional people who made this book possible. Most importantly, I thank Leah Zarra and the Skyhorse Publishing team for the opportunity to complete this project.

My thanks to John Watson of Imagemaker Photographic Studio, as always, for his incredible photography. His overall vision, tireless work ethic, and attention to detail continue to impress me in every one of our many shoots together.

A huge thank you to my mom, Angelika Hackett, for modelling the 50 exercises in this book, which involved a nine-hour photoshoot at the beach on a hot day in August. At almost seventy years old, she's twice my age—and has twice the energy! What an inspiration.

I'd like to acknowledge the four fitness coaches who contributed to this book: Emma Green, Jennifer Fidder, Ren Jones, and Melody Schoenfeld. Thank you for sharing your expertise with our readers.

Big thanks to my team who kept my business running while I worked on this book: Kaylin Foisy, Izzy Pope-Moore, Jess Peacock, and my coach colleague Zoe Peled. I'm lucky to be able to work with such extraordinary humans. Thank you also to our amazing clients all over the world, who inspire me in fitness (and in life) on a daily basis.

Thank you to my family for their continued support of all my projects: my husband, Murray Inkster; my parents, Robert and Angelika Hackett; and my sister, Melanie Hackett.

About the Author

Karina Inkster is a fitness coach, author, and podcast host. Vegan since 2003 and vegetarian since 1998, Karina's award-winning online programs offer plant-based fitness and nutrition coaching to clients around the world.

Karina's other books include *The Vegan Athlete: A Complete Guide to a Healthy, Plant-Based, Active Lifestyle*; *Resistance Band Workouts: 50 Exercises for Strength Training at Home or On the Go*; *Vegan Vitality: Your Complete Guide to a Healthy, Active, Plant-Based Lifestyle*; and *Foam Rolling: 50 Exercises for Massage, Injury Prevention, and Core Strength*. She's a writer for several magazines, and hosts the No-B.S. Vegan podcast. She holds a Master's degree in Gerontology, specializing in health and aging.

When she's not working with her clients, writing, or doing a ridiculous number of chin-ups, you'll find Karina playing accordion, piano, and Australian didgeridoo; hanging out with her two cats; or sneaking spinach into her husband's smoothies. Visit her website at karinainkster.com.